MATHÉMATIQUES

D1757686

3 0116 00499 5930

This book is due for return not later than the
last date stamped below, unless recalled sooner.

Habib Ammari

An Introduction to Mathematics of Emerging Biomedical Imaging

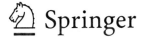 Springer

Habib Ammari

CNRS
Laboratoire Ondes et Acoustique
École Supérieure de Physique et de Chimie Industrielles (ESPCI)
10 Rue Vauquelin
75231 Paris Cedex 05
France

and

Centre de Mathématiques Appliquées
École Polytechnique
91128 Palaiseau Cedex
France
habib.ammari@espci.fr
habib.ammari@polytechnique.fr
www.cmap.polytechnique.fr/~ammari/

Library Congress Control Number: 2008921393

Mathematics Subject Classification (2000): 92C55, 31A25, 31A10, 35B25, 35J55, 35J65, 34A55

ISSN 1154-483X
ISBN 978-3-540-79552-0 Springer Berlin Heidelberg New York
e-ISBN 978-3-540-79553-7 Springer Berlin Heidelberg New York

Springer est membre du Springer Science+Business Media
©Springer-Verlag Berlin Heidelberg 2008
springer.com
WMXDesign GmbH

Imprimé sur papier non acide 3100/SPi - 5 4 3 2 1 0 -

Preface

This book has grown out of lecture notes for a course on mathematical methods in biomedical imaging at Ecole Polytechnique.

Biomedical imaging is a fascinating research area to applied mathematicians. It is quite a hot topic that appeals to many students. Challenging imaging problems arise and they often trigger the investigation of fundamental problems in various branches of mathematics (including inverse problems, PDEs, harmonic analysis, complex analysis, numerical analysis, optimization, image analysis). Many applied mathematicians have experienced a great feeling of accomplishment when they saw their work having a real impact on medical and clinical decision making.

In this book, we underscore the importance of mathematical aspects of emerging biomedical imaging. We acknowledge that biomedical technology has already had success in performing imaging in many different contexts, however in this book we highlight the most recent developments in emerging, non standard, techniques that are not yet established as standard imaging tools. The contents of this book introduce the reader to the basic mathematical concepts of biomathematical imaging and lay the ground for advanced issues in innovative techniques in the field.

This book may be used for a graduate-level course in applied mathematics and should help prepare the reader for a deeper understanding of research areas in biomedical imaging. Some background knowledge of PDEs is assumed.

I thank Frank Bauer, Natacha Béreux, Yves Capdeboscq, and Darko Volkov for reading an early version of this book and making a number of helpful suggestions. I am also indebted to Sylvain Baillet and Mickael Tanter for providing me with some of the illustrations presented in this book. Finally, I would like to acknowledge the support by the ANR project EchoScan (AN-06-Blan-0089).

Paris, June 2007   *Habib Ammari*

Contents

Introduction

Tomography is an important area in the ever-growing field of biomedical imaging science. The term *tomos* means cut in Greek, but tomography is concerned with creating images of the internal organization of an object without physically cutting it open. To a beginner, it might seem inconceivable, but as your reading of this book progresses, you will appreciate not only the feasibility but also the inherent beauty and simplicity of tomography.

The impact of tomographic imaging in diagnostic medicine has been revolutionary, since it has enabled doctors to view internal organs with unprecedented precision and safety to the patient. Biomedical imaging has seen truly exciting advances in recent years. These advances not only create new and better ways to extract information about our bodies, but they also offer the promise of making some imaging tools more convenient and economical.

The first medical application utilized X-rays for forming images of tissues based on their X-ray attenuation coefficient. X-rays are a form of electromagnetic radiation with a wavelength in the range of 10 to 0.01 nanometers. More recently, however, medical imaging has also been successfully accomplished with magnetic resonance (MRI), electrical impedance tomography (EIT), electrical and magnetic source imaging, ultrasound, microwaves and elastography; the imaged parameter being different in each case. Hybrid or multi-physics techniques including magnetic resonance electrical impedance tomography (MREIT), impediography, magnetic resonance elastography (MRE) are currently being researched. These very promising techniques are not yet established as standard imaging tools in biomedicine. They are still the subject of very active academic research. Future improvements in these exciting imaging techniques require continued research in the mathematical sciences, a field that has contributed greatly to biomedical imaging and will continue to do so.

Although these tomographic imaging modalities use different physical principles for signal generation and detection, the underlying mathematics are, to a large extent, the same. The tomographic imaging process essentially involves two transformations. The first transformation, often referred to as the imaging equation, governs how the experimental data are collected, and the second, often referred as the image reconstruction equation, determines how the measured data are processed for image formation. The first step is known as the forward problem and the second step is the so-called inverse problem. The imaging equations are derived as approximations to complex physical phenomena. A good formulation in terms of the tissue parameters relative to each modality is the basis of any attack on the corresponding inverse problem. Considerable effort should be spent producing increasingly realistic models that allow for effective numerical simulation and validation in terms of real data.

This book focuses on the mathematical methods for the image reconstruction problem. In imaging with magnetic resonance we wish to reconstruct the magnetic properties of the object. The problem can be set up as reconstructing an image from its projections. This is not the case when ultrasound waves or microwaves are used as energy sources; although the aim is the same as X-rays. The X-rays are non-diffracting, *i.e.*, they travel in straight lines, whereas ultrasound and microwaves are diffracting. When an object is illuminated with a diffracting source, the wave field is scattered practically in all directions. Both magnetic source imaging and electrical source imaging seek to determine the location, orientation, and magnitude of current sources within the body.

In this book we cover several aspects of tomography: tomography with non-diffracting sources, tomography with diffracting sources, and multi-physics approaches to tomographic imaging. The presentation is far from being complete. However, we emphasize the mathematical concepts and tools for image reconstruction. Its main focuses are, on one side, on promising anomaly detection techniques in EIT and in elastic imaging using the method of small volume expansions and, on the other side, on emerging multi-physics or hybrid imaging approaches (MREIT, impediography, MRE).

The book is organized as follows. Chapter 1 outlines the biomedical imaging modalities discussed in this book. Chapter 2 reviews some of the fundamental mathematical concepts that are key to understanding imaging principles. Chapter 3 collects some preliminary results regarding layer potentials. This chapter offers a comprehensive treatment of the subject of integral equations. Chapter 4 deals with the mathematical basis of tomography with non-diffracting sources. Two fundamental image reconstruction problems are discussed: (i) reconstruction from Fourier transform samples, and (ii) reconstruction from Radon transform samples. Chapter 5 is devoted to general algorithms in EIT and ultrasound imaging. Chapter 6 outlines electrical and magnetic source imaging reconstruction methods for focal brain activity. Chapter 7 covers the method of small volume expansions. Based on this method we provide in Chapter 6 robust and efficient algorithms for imaging small electrical and electromagnetic anomalies. Chapters 8 to 10 discuss emerging multi-physics approaches for imaging, namely MREIT, impediography, and MRE. The bibliography provides a list of relevant references. It is by no means comprehensive. However, it should provide the reader with some useful guidance in searching for further details on the main ideas and approaches discussed in this book.

1

Biomedical Imaging Modalities

The introduction of advanced imaging techniques has improved significantly the quality of medical care available to patients. Noninvasive imaging modalities allow a physician to make increasingly accurate diagnoses and render precise and measured modes of treatment. A multitude of imaging modalities are available currently or subject of active and promising research. This chapter outlines those discussed in this book.

1.1 X-Ray Imaging and Computed Tomography

X-ray imaging is a transmission-based technique in which X-rays from a source pass through the patient and are detected either by film or an ionization chamber on the opposite side of the body. Contrast in the image between different tissues arises from differential attenuation of X-rays in the body. For example, X-ray attenuation is particularly efficient in bone, but less so in soft tissues. In planar X-ray radiography, the image produced is a simple two-dimensional projection of the tissues lying between the X-ray source and the film. Planar X-ray radiography is used for example to study the liver and the abdomen and to detect diseases of the lung or broken ribs.

Planar X-ray radiography of overlapping layers of soft tissue or complex bone structures can often be difficult to interpret. In these cases, X-ray computed tomography (CT) is used. In CT, the X-ray source is tightly collimated to interrogate a thin slice through the patient. The source and detectors rotate together around the patient, producing a series of one-dimensional projections at a number of different angles. These data are reconstructed to give a two-dimensional image and provide a reasonable contrast between soft tissues. The mathematical basis for reconstruction of an image from a series of projections is the Radon transform. Recent developments in spiral and multi-slice CT have enabled the acquisition of full three-dimensional images in a single patient breath-hold.

The biggest disadvantage of both X-ray and CT imaging is the fact that the technique uses ionizing radiation. Because ionizing radiation can cause tissue damage, there is a limit on the total radiation dose per year to which a patient can be exposed. Radiation dose is of particular concern in pediatric and obstetric radiology. Figure 1.1 shows an X-ray image of breast cancer.

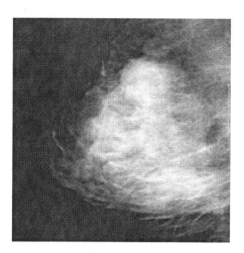

Fig. 1.1. X-ray image of breast cancer.

1.2 Magnetic Resonance Imaging

Magnetic resonance imaging (MRI) is a non-ionizing technique with full three-dimensional capabilities, excellent soft-tissue contrast, and high spatial resolution (about 1mm). In general, the temporal resolution is much slower than for computed tomography, with scans typically lasting between 3 and 10 min, and MRI is therefore much more susceptible to patient motion. The cost of MRI scanners is relatively high, with the price of a typical clinical 1.5-T whole-body imager on the order of 1 million euros. The major uses of MRI are in the areas of assessing brain disease, spinal disorders, cardiac function, and musculoskeletal damage.

The MRI signal arises from protons in the body, primarily water, but also lipid. The patient is placed inside a strong magnet, which produces a static magnetic field typically more than 10^4 times stronger than the earth's magnetic field. Each proton, being a charged particle with angular momentum, can be considered as acting as a small magnet. The protons align in two configurations, with their internal magnetic fields aligned either parallel or anti-parallel to the direction of the large static magnetic field. The protons process around the direction of the static magnetic field. The frequency of precession is proportional to the strength of the static magnetic field. Application of a weak radio-frequency field causes the protons to process coherently, and the sum of all the protons precessing is detected as an induced voltage in a tuned detector coil.

Spatial information is encoded into the image using magnetic field gradient. These impose a linear variation in all three dimensions in the magnetic field present within the patient. As a result of these variations, the precessional frequencies of the protons are also linearly dependent upon their spatial location. The frequency and the phase of the precessing magnetization is measured by the radio-frequency coil, and the analog signal is digitized. An inverse two-dimensional Fourier transform is performed to convert the signal into the spatial domain to produce the image. By varying the data acquisition parameters, differential contrast between soft tissues can be introduced with high spatial resolution. Figure 1.2 shows an MRI image of breast cancer. MRI has high sensitivity but low specificity. It is not capable of discriminating benign from malignant lesions.

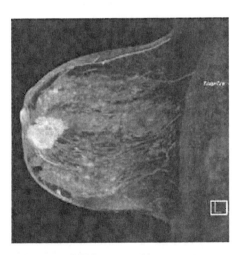

Fig. 1.2. MRI image of breast cancer.

1.3 Electrical Impedance Tomography

Electrical impedance tomography (EIT) uses low-frequency electrical current to probe a body; the method is sensitive to changes in electrical conductivity. By injecting known amounts of current and measuring the resulting electrical potential field at points on the boundary of the body, it is possible to "invert" such data to determine the conductivity or resistivity of the region of the body probed by the currents. This method can also be used in principle to image changes in dielectric constant at higher frequencies, which is why the method is often called "impedance" tomography rather than "conductivity" or "resistivity" tomography. However, the aspect of the method that is most fully developed to date is the imaging of conductivity/resistivity. Potential applications of EIT include determination of cardiac output, monitoring for pulmonary edema, and screening for breast cancer.

There is a formal mathematical analogy between EIT and CT, since in either case data must be processed to produce the desired image of interior structure and, furthermore, the imaging is often performed on two-dimensional slices through the body. EIT uses diffusion of current to deduce conductivity distribution, unlike MRI and CT.

EIT is expected to have relatively poor resolution compared to MRI, and CT. However, at the present time, EIT is the only method known that images electrical conductivity, although MRI and electromagnetic methods also have some potential to measure conductivity. So, for applications requiring knowledge of the distribution of this parameter through a body, EIT is an important method to consider for medical imaging, regardless of its resolving power.

On the other hand, EIT has some very attractive features. The technology for doing electrical impedance imaging is safe and inexpensive, and therefore could be made available at multiple locations (for example, at bedside) in hospitals. At the low current levels needed for this imaging technique, the method is not known to cause any long-term harm to the patient, and therefore could be used to do continuous (or frequent, but intermittent) monitoring of bedridden patients.

The impedance imaging problem is nonlinear and extremely ill posed, which means that large changes in interior properties can result in only small changes in the measurements. The classical image reconstruction algorithms view EIT as an optimization problem. An initial conductivity distribution is iteratively updated, so as to minimize in the least-squares sense the difference between measured and computed boundary voltages. This approach is quite greedy in computational time, yet produces images with deceivingly poor accuracy and spatial resolution.

In the 1980's, Barber and Brown introduced a back-projection algorithm, that was the first fast and efficient algorithm for EIT, although it provides images with very low resolution. Since this algorithm is inspired from computed tomography, it can be viewed as a generalized Radon transform method.

A third technique is dynamical electrical impedance imaging to produce images of changes in conductivity due to cardiac or respiratory functions. Its main idea consists in viewing the conductivity as the sum of a static term plus a perturbation. The mathematical problem here is to visualize the perturbation term by an EIT system. Although this algorithm provides accurate images if the initial guess of the background conductivity is good, its resolution does not completely satisfy practitioners especially when screening for breast cancer.

1.4 T-Scan Electrical Impedance Imaging System for Anomaly Detection

Recently, a commercial system called TransScan TS2000 (TransScan Medical, Ltd, Migdal Ha'Emek, Israel) has been released for adjunctive clinical uses with X-ray mammography in the diagnostic of breast cancer. Interestingly, the TransScan system is similar to the frontal plane impedance camera that initiated EIT research early in 1978. The mathematical model of the TransScan can be viewed as a realistic or practical version of the general EIT system, so any theory developed for this model can be applied to other areas in EIT, especially to detection of anomalies. In the TransScan, a patient holds a metallic cylindrical reference electrode, through which a constant voltage of 1 to 2.5 V, with frequencies spanning 100 Hz-100 KHz, is applied. A scanning probe with a planar array of electrodes, kept at ground potential, is placed on the breast. The voltage difference between the hand and the probe induces a current flow through the breast, from which information about the impedance distribution in the breast can be extracted. See Fig. 1.3

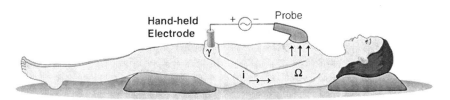

Fig. 1.3. Tscan.

1.5 Electrical and Magnetic Source Imaging

Electrical source imaging (ESI) is an emerging technique for reconstructing brain or cardiac electrical activity from electrical potentials measured away from the brain or heart. The concept of ESI is to improve on electroencephalography (EEG) or electrocardiography (ECG) by determining the locations of sources of current in the body from measurements of voltages. ESI could improve diagnoses and guide therapy related to epilepsy and heart conduction abnormalities through its capability for locating an electrical abnormality that is to be removed. Differences in potential within the brain, heart, and other tissues reflect the segregation of electrical charges at certain locations within these three-dimensional conductors as nerves are excited, causing cell membrane potentials to change. While the potential measured at some distance from an electrical charge generally decreases with increasing distance, the situation is more complex within the body; generators of the EEG, for example, are not simple point-like charge accumulations but rather are dipole-like layers. Moreover, these layers are convoluted and enmeshed in a volume conductor with spatially heterogeneous conductivity. The particular geometry and orientation of these layers determines the potential distribution within or at the surface of the body. The classical approach to studying brain electrical activity involves recognizing patterns in a set of waveforms showing voltage as a function of time, acquired from about 20 electrodes placed on the scalp. While frequency analysis methods can indicate probable Alzheimer's disease by the abnormal distribution of spatial frequency bands true distribution of neuronal activity, knowledge of which could lead to more refined diagnoses, is masked or blurred by the conducting tissue layers between the central cortex and the electrodes. Cardiac electrical activity is likewise spatially complex, and involves the propagation of excitation wave fronts in the heart. Standard electrocardiographic techniques such as electrocardiography (ECG) and vectorcardiography (VCG) are very limited in their ability to provide information on regional electrical activity and to localize bioelectrical events in the heart. In fact, VCG lumps all cardiac wave fronts into a single dipole located at the center of the heart and known as the heart vector. Traditional ECG and VCG employ a small number of electrodes to measure potentials from the body surface, and the patterns of electrical activity cannot give the information required for characterizing the electrical activity of the heart. Non-invasive electrocardiography requires simultaneous recordings of electrical potential from 100 to 250 torso sites in order to map the body surface potential. These body surface potential maps (BSPMs) reflect the regional time course of electrical activity of the heart, information that is important for clinical treatment. Body surface potential distribution is a very low resolution projection of cardiac electrical activity, and details of regional electrical activity in the heart cannot be determined merely from visual inspection of the BSPMs. A mathematical method of reconstructing endocardial potentials is greatly needed.

Ion currents arising in the neurons of the heart and the brain produce magnetic fields outside the body that can be measured by arrays of SQUID (superconducting quantum interference device) detectors placed near the chest or head; the recording of these magnetic fields is known as magnetocardiography (MCG) or magnetoencephalography (MEG). Magnetic source imaging (MSI) is the reconstruction of the current sources in the heart or brain from these recorded magnetic fields. These fields result from the synchronous activity of tens or hundreds of thousands of neurons. Both magnetic source imaging and electrical source imaging seek to determine the location, orientation, and magnitude of current sources within the body. The magnetic field at the surface is most strongly determined by current sources directed parallel to the surface, but the electrical potentials are determined by current sources directed perpendicular to the surface. Other than the signal distortion from the heterogeneity of tissue conductivity, there is no clear physical reason that the clinical information produced by biomagnetic measurements could not as well be obtained from electrical potential mapping. An advantage of MSI over ESI is that all body tissues are magnetically transparent and the magnetic fields propagate to the surface without distortion. The electrical potentials at the surface, on the other hand, are distorted by variations in conductivity within the body; this is especially true in the head, where the low conductivity of the skull both distorts and hides the electrical activity of the brain. A disadvantage of MSI is that the need for cryogenic cooling and a magnetically shielded room makes the procedure cumbersome with the present technology.

Biomagnetic source imaging offers a tool to study processes where electrical function is important. Promising results have been obtained in the fields of cardiology and epilepsy. An exciting research on challenging signal processing issues for EEG and MEG data analysis is being conducted at Laboratoire de Neurosciences Cognitives & Imagerie Cérébrale in Paris (http://cogimage.dsi.cnrs.fr/index.htm). A comprehensive set of tools dedicated to MEG and EEG data visualization and processing is available at http://neuroimage.usc.edu/brainstorm/. Figure 1.4 shows a MEG imaging system and a MEG reconstruction of electrical brain activity coherent with the speed of hand movements.

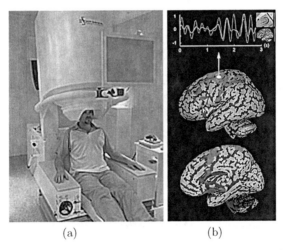

(a)   (b)

Fig. 1.4. (a) MEG imaging system; (b) Electrical brain activity coherent with the speed of hand movements.

1.6 Magnetic Resonance Electrical Impedance Tomography

Since all the present EIT technologies are only practically applicable in feature extraction of anomalies, improving EIT calls for innovative measurement techniques that incorporate structural information. A very promising direction of research is the recent magnetic resonance imaging technique, called current density imaging, which measures the internal current density distribution.

When one injects a current into a subject, it produces a magnetic field as well as an electric field. In EIT, one utilizes only the electrical quantities. Furthermore, since there is no noninvasive way of getting measurements of electrical quantities from inside the subject, we are limited in EIT by the boundary current-voltage data which is insensitive to internal conductivity perturbations. Using a magnetic resonance imaging scanner, one can enrich the EIT data by measuring the internal magnetic flux density. This technique called magnetic resonance current magnetic resonance electrical impedance tomography (MREIT) perceives the distortion of current pathways due to the conductivity distribution to be imaged and overcomes the severe ill-posedness character of EIT. It provides high-resolution conductivity images. However, it has a number of disadvantages, among which the lack of portability and a potentially long imaging time. Moreover, it uses an expensive magnetic resonance imaging scanner.

MREIT has been developed at the Impedance Imaging Research Center in Seoul (http://iirc.khu.ac.kr/). See Fig. 1.5.

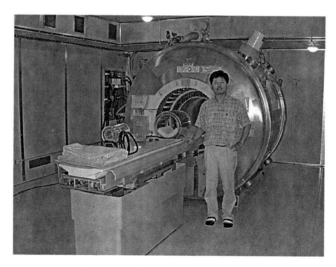

Fig. 1.5. MREIT imaging system.

1.7 Impediography

Another mathematical direction for future EIT research in view of biomedical applications, without eliminating the most important merits of EIT (real time imaging, low cost, portability). The method named impediography is based on the simultaneous measurement of an electric current and of acoustic vibrations induced by ultrasound waves. The core idea of impediography is to extract more information about the conductivity from data that has been enriched by coupling the electric measurements to localized elastic perturbations. Its intrinsic resolution depends on the size of the focal spot of the acoustic perturbation, and thus it provides high resolution images.

Impediography is being developed at Laboratoire Ondes et Acoustique (LOA) in Paris (http://www.espci.loa.fr).

1.8 Ultrasound Imaging

Ultrasound imaging is a noninvasive, easily portable, and relatively inexpensive diagnostic modality which finds extensive use in the clinic. The major clinical applications of ultrasound include many aspects of obstetrics and gynecology involving the assessment of fetal health, intra-abdominal imaging of the liver, kidney, and the detection of compromised blood flow in veins and arteries.

Operating typically at frequencies between 1 and 10 MHz, ultrasound imaging produces images via the backscattering of mechanical energy from interfaces between tissues and small structures within tissue. It has high spatial resolution, particularly at high frequencies, and involves no ionizing radiation. The weakness of the technique include the relatively poor soft-tissue contrast and the fact that gas and bone impede the passage of ultrasound waves, meaning that certain organs can not easily be imaged. Figure 1.6 shows an ultrasound probe and an ultrasound image of breast cancer. Compared to Fig. 1.2, it is with much lower sensitivity.

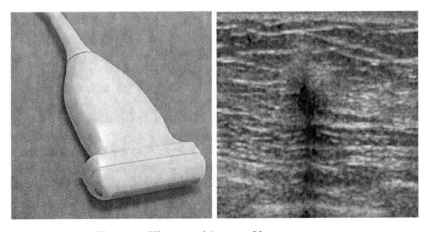

Fig. 1.6. Ultrasound image of breast cancer.

1.9 Microwave Imaging

Ultrasound specificity in breast cancer characterization is low as a result of the overlapping acoustic characteristics of benign and malignant lesions. Recently, microwave imaging is emerging as a new promising modality for the detection of breast cancer because of the high electrical contrasts between malignant tumors and normal breast tissue. Microwaves interact with biological tissues primarily according to the tissue water content, a fundamentally different mechanism from ultrasound. Due to the high vascular content or water content related to tumor angiogenesis, malignant tumors have significantly larger microwave scattering cross sections than normal fatty breast tissues.

1.10 Elastic Imaging

The mechanical properties of soft tissues are important indicators for biomedical research and diagnosis since they are generally correlated with the tissue pathological changes. Although different in terms of elastic stiffness, some tumors are not readily detectable by conventional imaging modalities such as CT, ultrasound imaging, and MRI. Palpation is frequently used to find firm lesions. However, deep lesions in large breasts may not be palpable until they grow large and become incurable. Recognizing that the elastic modulus stiffness change of tissues could indicate the tissue pathological evolution, elastic imaging was developed to detect and characterize tumors by combining some forms of tissue excitation techniques with methods for detection of tissue response.

1.11 Magnetic Resonance Elastography

Magnetic resonance elastography (MRE) is a recently developed technique that can directly visualize and quantitatively measure propagating acoustic strain waves in tissue-like materials subjected to harmonic mechanical excitation. Elastic waves at frequencies in the 10–1000 Hz range are used as a probe because they are much less attenuated than at higher frequencies, their wavelength in tissue-like materials is in the useful range of millimeters to tens of millimeters. A phase-contrast MRI technique is used to spatially map and measure the wave displacement patterns. From these data, local quantitative values of shear modulus can be calculated and images that depict tissue elasticity or stiffness can be generated. Very active research on MRE is being conducted at LOA. See Fig. 1.7.

It is worth pointing out that impediography, MREIT, and MRE are not yet established as standard imaging tools in medicine, and that they are still the subject of mainly academic research.

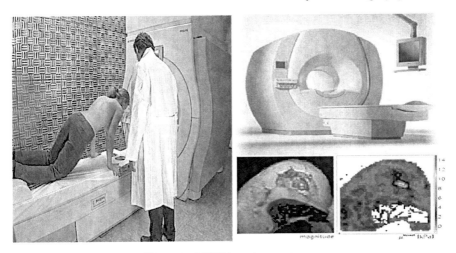

Fig. 1.7. MRE imaging system.

1.12 Optical Tomography

Optical tomography is a new technique being developed to estimate the optical properties of the body. It is based on the discovery that human tissue has a relative transparency to infra red light in the region 700-1000nm over the highly attenuated visible spectrum. Its principle is to use multiple movable light sources and detectors attached to the tissue surface to collect information on light attenuation, and to reconstruct the internal absorption and scattering distributions. Unusual growths inside the tissue may be discerned from the recovered optical densities because tumorous tissue has different scattering and absorption properties.

Applications of this emerging imaging technique also include a monitoring of cerebral blood and tissue oxygenation of newborn infants and functional mapping of brain activation during physical or mental exercise.

The most comprehensive mathematical model for optical tomography is the radiation transfer equation for the particle flux. When the tissue is strongly scattering, the signal propagation in the medium is diffuse and the particle flux is essentially isotropic a small distance away from the sources. In this case, the diffusion approximation can be used.

Single photon emission computed tomography (SPECT) and positron emission tomography (PET) are not discussed in this book.

Part I

Mathematical Tools

2

Preliminaries

This chapter reviews some mathematical concepts essential for understanding biomedical imaging principles. We first review commonly used special functions, functional spaces, and two integral transforms: the Fourier transform and the Radon transform. We then collect basic facts about the Moore-Penrose generalized inverse, singular value decomposition, and compact operators. The theory of regularization of ill-posed inverse problems is briefly discussed. The final section examines image characteristics with respect to various data acquisition and processing schemes. We focus specifically on issues related to image resolution, signal-to-noise ratio, and image artifacts.

2.1 Special Functions

Bessel functions of the first kind of real order ν, denoted by $J_\nu(x)$, are useful for describing some imaging effects. One definition of $J_\nu(x)$ is given in terms of the series representation

$$J_\nu(x) = (\frac{x}{2})^\nu \sum_{l=0}^{+\infty} \frac{(-x^2/4)^l}{l!\Gamma(\nu+l+1)} , \qquad (2.1)$$

where the gamma function Γ is defined by

$$\Gamma(z) = \int_0^{+\infty} e^{-t} t^{z-1} \, dt \quad \text{for } \Re e(z) > 0.$$

Another formula, valid for $\Re e\, \nu > -\frac{1}{2}$, is

$$J_\nu(x) = [\Gamma(\frac{1}{2})\Gamma(\nu+\frac{1}{2})]^{-1}(\frac{x}{2})^\nu \int_{-1}^{1} (1-t^2)^{\nu-\frac{1}{2}} e^{ixt} \, dt. \qquad (2.2)$$

Some useful identities for Bessel functions are summarized below. For further details, we refer the reader to [118, pages 225–233].

We have the recurrence relation

$$\left(\frac{d}{dx} + \frac{\nu}{x}\right)J_\nu(x) = J_{\nu-1}(x) . \tag{2.3}$$

For $n \in \mathbb{Z}$, we have the integral representation

$$J_n(x) = \frac{1}{2\pi} \int_{-\pi}^{\pi} e^{ix \sin \phi - in\phi} d\phi ,$$

i.e., the functions $J_n(x)$ are the Fourier coefficients of $e^{ix \sin \phi}$. Therefore

$$e^{ix \sin \phi} = \sum_{n \in \mathbb{Z}} J_n(x)e^{in\phi} . \tag{2.4}$$

By the principle of analytic continuation, formula (2.4) is even valid for all complex ϕ. See Fig. 2.1 where J_n for $n = 0, \ldots, 5$ are plotted.

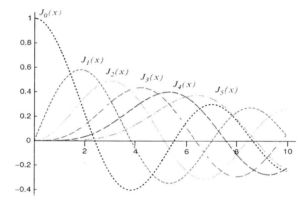

Fig. 2.1. Plots of Bessel functions $J_n(x), n = 0, \ldots, 5$.

For arguments $x < \nu$, the Bessel functions look qualitatively like simple powers law, with the asymptotic form for $0 < x \ll \nu$

$$J_\nu(x) \sim \frac{1}{\Gamma(\nu + 1)} \left(\frac{x}{2}\right)^\nu .$$

For $x > \nu$, the Bessel functions look qualitatively like cosine waves whose amplitude decay as $x^{-1/2}$. The asymptotic form for $x \gg \nu$ is

$$J_\nu(x) \sim \sqrt{\frac{2}{\pi x}} \cos \left(x - \frac{\nu\pi}{2} - \frac{\pi}{4}\right) .$$

In the transition region where $x \sim \nu$, the typical amplitude of the Bessel functions is

$$J_\nu(\nu) \sim \frac{2^{1/3}}{3^{2/3}\Gamma\left(\frac{2}{3}\right)} \frac{1}{\nu^{1/3}} \sim \frac{0.4473}{\nu^{1/3}} \ ,$$

which holds asymptotically for large ν.

The Bessel function J_ν solves the ODE, known as Bessel's equation

$$\left(\frac{d^2}{dx^2} + \frac{1}{x}\frac{d}{dx} + \left(1 - \frac{\nu^2}{x^2}\right)\right) J_\nu(x) = 0 \ , \tag{2.5}$$

or equivalently,

$$(\frac{d}{dx} - \frac{\nu-1}{x})(\frac{d}{dx} + \frac{\nu}{x})J_\nu(x) = -J_\nu(x) \ . \tag{2.6}$$

Note that adding and subtracting (2.3) and (2.6) produce the identities

$$2J'_\nu(x) = J_{\nu-1}(x) - J_{\nu+1}(x) \ ,$$
$$\frac{2\nu}{x}J_\nu(x) = J_{\nu-1}(x) + J_{\nu+1}(x) \ .$$

Equation (2.5), for each ν, has a two-dimensional solution space. Note that $J_{-\nu}$ is also a solution. From the expression (2.1) it is clear that J_ν and $J_{-\nu}$ are linearly independent provided ν is not an integer. On the other hand, comparison of power series shows

$$J_{-n}(x) = (-1)^n J_n(x), \quad n \in \mathbb{N} \ .$$

A calculation of the Wronskian shows that

$$W(J_\nu, J_{-\nu})(x) = -2\frac{\sin \pi\nu}{\pi x} \ .$$

Therefore, J_ν and $J_{-\nu}$ are linearly independent, and consequently they form a basis of solutions to (2.5), if and only if ν is not an integer. To construct a basis of solutions uniformly good for all ν, it is natural to set

$$Y_\nu(x) = \frac{J_\nu(x)\cos \pi\nu - J_{-\nu}(x)}{\sin \pi\nu} \tag{2.7}$$

when ν is not an integer, and define

$$Y_n(x) = \lim_{\nu \to n} Y_\nu(x) \ .$$

We have

$$W(J_\nu, Y_\nu)(x) = \frac{2}{\pi x} \ ,$$

for all ν. Another important pair of solutions to Bessel's equation is the pair of Hankel functions

$$H_\nu^{(1)}(x) = J_\nu(x) + iY_\nu(x), \quad H_\nu^{(1)}(x) = J_\nu(x) - iY_\nu(x) \ .$$

It is worth pointing out that the Bessel functions $J_{n+1/2}(x)$, for n an integer, are elementary functions. For $\nu = n + 1/2$, the integrand in (2.2) involves $(1 - t^2)^n$, so the integral can be evaluated explicitly. We have, in particular,

$$J_{1/2}(x) = (\frac{2}{\pi x})^{1/2} \sin x .$$

Then (2.3) gives

$$J_{-1/2}(x) = (\frac{2}{\pi x})^{1/2} \cos x ,$$

which by (2.7) is equal to $-Y_{1/2}(x)$. Applying (2.6) and (2.3) repeatedly gives

$$J_{n+1/2}(x) = (-1)^n \prod_{l=1}^{n} (\frac{d}{dx} - \frac{l - \frac{1}{2}}{x}) \frac{\sin x}{\sqrt{2\pi x}}$$

and the same sort of formula for $J_{-n-1/2}(x)$, with the $(-1)^n$ removed, and $\sin x$ replaced by $\cos x$.

The functions

$$j_n(x) := \sqrt{\frac{\pi}{2}} \frac{J_{n+\frac{1}{2}}(x)}{\sqrt{x}} ,$$

and

$$y_n(x) := \sqrt{\frac{\pi}{2}} \frac{Y_{n+\frac{1}{2}}(x)}{\sqrt{x}}$$

are known as the spherical Bessel functions and form a basis for the solution space of the spherical Bessel equation

$$\left(\frac{d^2}{dx^2} + \frac{1}{x} \frac{d}{dx} + (1 - \frac{n(n+1)}{x^2}) \right) f(x) = 0 .$$

2.2 Sobolev Spaces

For ease of notation we will sometimes use ∂ and ∂^2 to denote the gradient and the Hessian, respectively.

Let D be a bounded smooth domain. We define the Banach spaces $W^{1,p}(D), 1 < p < +\infty$, by

$$W^{1,p}(D) = \left\{ u \in L^p(D) : \int_D |u|^p + \int_D |\nabla u|^p < +\infty \right\} ,$$

where ∇u is interpreted as a distribution, and $L^p(D)$ is defined in the usual way, with

$$\|u\|_{L^p(D)} = \left(\int_D |u|^p \right)^{1/p} .$$

The space $W^{1,p}(D)$ is equipped with the norm

$$\|u\|_{W^{1,p}(D)} = \left(\int_D |u|^p + \int_D |\nabla u|^p \right)^{1/p} .$$

Another Banach space $W_0^{1,p}(D)$ arises by taking the closure of $\mathcal{C}_0^\infty(D)$, the set of infinitely differentiable functions with compact support in D, in $W^{1,p}(D)$. The spaces $W^{1,p}(D)$ and $W_0^{1,p}(D)$ do not coincide for bounded D. The case $p = 2$ is special, since the spaces $W^{1,2}(D)$ and $W_0^{1,2}(D)$ are Hilbert spaces under the scalar product

$$(u, v) = \int_D u\,v + \int_D \nabla u \cdot \nabla v .$$

We will also need the space $W_{\mathrm{loc}}^{1,2}(\mathbb{R}^d \setminus \overline{D})$ of functions $u \in L_{\mathrm{loc}}^2(\mathbb{R}^d \setminus \overline{D})$, the set of locally square summable functions in $\mathbb{R}^d \setminus \overline{D}$, such that

$$hu \in W^{1,2}(\mathbb{R}^d \setminus \overline{D}), \forall\, h \in \mathcal{C}_0^\infty(\mathbb{R}^d \setminus \overline{D}) .$$

Further, we define $W^{2,2}(D)$ as the space of functions $u \in W^{1,2}(D)$ such that $\partial^2 u \in L^2(D)$ and the space $W^{3/2,2}(D)$ as the interpolation space $[W^{1,2}(D), W^{2,2}(D)]_{1/2}$.

It is known that the trace operator $u \mapsto u|_{\partial D}$ is a bounded linear surjective operator from $W^{1,2}(D)$ into $W_{\frac{1}{2}}^2(\partial D)$, where $f \in W_{\frac{1}{2}}^2(\partial D)$ if and only if $f \in L^2(\partial D)$ and

$$\int_{\partial D} \int_{\partial D} \frac{|f(x) - f(y)|^2}{|x - y|^d}\, d\sigma(x)\, d\sigma(y) < +\infty .$$

We set $W_{-\frac{1}{2}}^2(\partial D) = (W_{\frac{1}{2}}^2(\partial D))^*$ and let $\langle,\rangle_{\frac{1}{2}, -\frac{1}{2}}$ denote the duality pair between these dual spaces.

Finally, let $T_1, \ldots, T_{d-1}$ be an orthonormal basis for the tangent plane to ∂D at x and let

$$\partial/\partial T = \sum_{p=1}^{d-1} (\partial/\partial T_p)\, T_p$$

denote the tangential derivative on ∂D. We say that $f \in W_1^2(\partial D)$ if $f \in L^2(\partial D)$ and $\partial f/\partial T \in L^2(\partial D)$.

2.3 Fourier Analysis

The Fourier transform plays an important role in imaging. For $f \in L^1(\mathbb{R}^d)$, the Fourier transform $\mathcal{F}(f)$ and the inverse Fourier transform $\mathcal{F}^{-1}(f)$ are defined by

$$\mathcal{F}(f) \quad = (2\pi)^{-d/2} \int_{\mathbb{R}^d} e^{-ix\cdot\xi} f(x)\, dx\ ,$$

$$\mathcal{F}^{-1}(f) = (2\pi)^{-d/2} \int_{\mathbb{R}^d} e^{ix\cdot\xi} f(x)\, dx\ .$$

We use both transforms for other functions f, such as for functions in $L^2(\mathbb{R}^d)$ and even for the tempered distributions $\mathcal{S}'(\mathbb{R}^d)$, the dual of the Schwartz space of rapidly decreasing functions:

$$\mathcal{S}(\mathbb{R}^d) = \left\{ u \in \mathcal{C}^\infty(\mathbb{R}^d) : x^\beta D^\alpha u \in L^\infty(\mathbb{R}^d) \text{ for all } \alpha, \beta \ge 0 \right\},$$

where $x^\beta = x_1^{\beta_1} \dots x_d^{\beta_d}$, $D^\alpha = D_1^{\alpha_1} \dots D_d^{\alpha_d}$, with $D_j = -i\partial/\partial x_j$.

We list a few properties of the Fourier transform. It is easy to verify that $\mathcal{F} : \mathcal{S}(\mathbb{R}^d) \to \mathcal{S}(\mathbb{R}^d)$ and

$$\xi^\alpha D_\xi^\beta \mathcal{F}(f)(\xi) = (-1)^{|\beta|} \mathcal{F}(D^\alpha x^\beta f)(\xi)\ .$$

If $f_r(x) = f(rx), r > 0$, we have

$$\mathcal{F}(f_r)(\xi) = r^{-d} \mathcal{F}(f)(r^{-1}\xi)\ .$$

Likewise, if $f_y(x) = f(x + y)$ for $y \in \mathbb{R}^d$, then

$$\mathcal{F}(f_y)(\xi) = e^{i\xi\cdot y} \mathcal{F}(f)(\xi)\ .$$

We have the inversion formula: $\mathcal{F}\mathcal{F}^{-1} = \mathcal{F}^{-1}\mathcal{F} = I$ on both $\mathcal{S}(\mathbb{R}^d)$ and $\mathcal{S}'(\mathbb{R}^d)$. If $f \in L^2(\mathbb{R}^d)$, then $\mathcal{F}(f) \in L^2(\mathbb{R}^d)$, too. Plancherel's theorem says that $\mathcal{F} : L^2(\mathbb{R}^d) \to L^2(\mathbb{R}^d)$ is unitary, with inverse $\mathcal{F}^{-1}$.

If $f, g \in L^2(\mathbb{R}^d)$, then we have Parseval's relation:

$$\int_{\mathbb{R}^d} \mathcal{F}(f) g\, dx = \int_{\mathbb{R}^d} f \mathcal{F}(g)\, dx\ .$$

Since $\mathcal{F}^{-1}(\overline{f}) = \overline{\mathcal{F}(f)}$, these relations have their counterpart for $\mathcal{F}^{-1}$.

We now make some comments on the relation between the Fourier transform and convolutions. For $f \in \mathcal{S}'(\mathbb{R}^d), g \in \mathcal{S}(\mathbb{R}^d)$, the convolution

$$(f \star g)(x) = \int_{\mathbb{R}^d} f(x - y) g(y)\, dy$$

is defined, and we have

$$\mathcal{F}(f \star g) = (2\pi)^{d/2} \mathcal{F}(f)\mathcal{F}(g), \quad \mathcal{F}(fg) = (2\pi)^{-d/2} \mathcal{F}(f) \star \mathcal{F}(g)\ .$$

We need a few special Fourier transforms. For h a Gaussian function,

$$h(x) := e^{-|x|^2/2}, \quad x \in \mathbb{R}^d\ ,$$

we have

$$\mathcal{F}(h)(\xi) = e^{-|\xi|^2/2}, \quad \xi \in \mathbb{R}^d . \tag{2.8}$$

For δ_0 the Dirac function at the origin, i.e., $\delta_0 \in \mathcal{S}'(\mathbb{R}^d)$ and $\delta_0 f = f(0)$ for $f \in \mathcal{S}(\mathbb{R}^d)$, we have

$$\mathcal{F}(\delta_0) = (2\pi)^{-d/2} .$$

An approximation $\tilde{\delta}_K$ to δ_0 can be defined by

$$\mathcal{F}(\tilde{\delta}_K)(\xi) = \begin{cases} (2\pi)^{-d/2}, & |\xi| < K , \\ 0, & |\xi| \geq K . \end{cases}$$

We obtain

$$\tilde{\delta}_K(x) = (2\pi)^{-d/2} \frac{J_{d/2}(K|x|)}{(K|x|)^{d/2}} ,$$

where $J_{d/2}$ is the Bessel function of the first kind of order $d/2$.

One useful result is the classification of distributions supported at a single point. If $f \in \mathcal{S}'(\mathbb{R}^d)$ is supported by $\{0\}$, then there exist an integer n and complex numbers a_α such that

$$f = \sum_{|\alpha| \leq n} a_\alpha D^\alpha \delta_0 .$$

The shah distribution

$$\text{shah}_K = \sum_{l \in \mathbb{Z}^d} \delta_{Kl} ,$$

where $\delta_y f = f(y)$, has the Fourier transform

$$\mathcal{F}(\text{shah}_{2\pi/K}) = (2\pi)^{-d/2} K^d \text{shah}_K .$$

This is Poisson's formula. More generally, we have for $f \in \mathcal{S}(\mathbb{R}^d)$

$$\sum_{l \in \mathbb{Z}^d} \mathcal{F}(f)(\xi - \frac{2\pi l}{K}) = (2\pi)^{-d/2} K^d \sum_{l \in \mathbb{Z}^d} f(Kl) e^{-iK\xi \cdot l} . \tag{2.9}$$

2.3.1 Shannon's Sampling Theorem

We call a function (or distribution) in $\mathbb{R}^d, d \geq 1$, whose Fourier transform vanishes outside $|\xi| \leq K$ band-limited with bandwidth K. Shannon's sampling theorem is the following. The reader is referred to [94, page 41] for a proof.

Theorem 2.3.1 (Shannon's Sampling Theorem) *Let $f \in L^2(\mathbb{R})$ be band-limited with bandwidth K, and let $0 < \Delta x \leq \pi/K$. Then f is uniquely determined by the values $f(l\Delta x), l \in \mathbb{Z}$. The smallest detail represented by such a function is then of size $2\pi/K$. We also have the explicit formula*

$$f(x) = \sum_{l \in \mathbb{Z}} f\left(\frac{l\pi}{K}\right) \frac{\sin(Kx - l\pi)}{Kx - l\pi} . \tag{2.10}$$

The sampling interval π/K is often imposed by computation or storage constraints and the support of $\mathcal{F}(f)$ is generally not included in $[-K, K]$. In this case the interpolation formula (2.10) does not recover f. We give a filtering procedure to reduce the resulting error, known as the aliasing artifact.

To apply Shannon's sampling theorem, f is approximated by the closest function $\tilde{f}$ whose Fourier transform has a support in $[-K, K]$. Plancherel's theorem proves that

$$
||f - \tilde{f}||^2 = \int_{-\infty}^{+\infty} |\mathcal{F}(f)(\xi) - \mathcal{F}(\tilde{f})(\xi)|^2 \, d\xi
$$

$$
= \int_{|\xi|>K} |\mathcal{F}(f)(\xi)|^2 \, d\xi + \int_{|\xi|<K} |\mathcal{F}(f)(\xi) - \mathcal{F}(\tilde{f})(\xi)|^2 \, d\xi \, .
$$

The distance is minimum when the second integral is zero and hence

$$
\mathcal{F}(\tilde{f})(\xi) = \mathcal{F}(f)(\xi)\chi([-K, K])(\xi) = \sqrt{2\pi}\mathcal{F}(\tilde{\delta}_K)(\xi)\mathcal{F}(f)(\xi) \, ,
$$

where $\chi([-K, K])$ is the characteristic function of the interval $[-K, K]$. This corresponds to $\tilde{f} = f \star \tilde{\delta}_K$. The filtering of $f(x)$ by $\tilde{\delta}_K(x) = \sin(K|x|)/(\pi K|x|)$ remove any frequency larger than K. Since $\mathcal{F}(\tilde{f})$ has a support in $[-K, K]$, the sampling theorem proves that $\tilde{f}$ can be recovered from the samples $\tilde{f}(l\pi/K)$.

In the two-dimensional case, we use the separable extension principle. This not only simplifies the mathematics but also leads to faster numerical algorithms along the rows and columns of images. If $\mathcal{F}(f)$ has a support included in $[-K_1, K_1] \times [-K_2, K_2]$ then the following two-dimensional sampling formula holds:

$$
f(x, y) = \sum_{l=(l_1, l_2)\in\mathbb{Z}^2} f\left(\frac{l_1\pi}{K_1}, \frac{l_2\pi}{K_2}\right) \frac{\sin(K_1 x - l_1\pi)}{K_1 x - l_1\pi} \frac{\sin(K_2 y - l_2\pi)}{K_2 y - l_2\pi} \, . \quad (2.11)
$$

If the support of $\mathcal{F}(f)$ is not included in the low-frequency rectangle $[-K_1, K_1] \times [-K_2, K_2]$ then we have to filter f with the low-pass separable filter $\tilde{\delta}_{K_1}(x) \, \tilde{\delta}_{K_2}(y)$.

2.3.2 Fast Fourier Transform

In tomography fast Fourier transform techniques (denoted FFT) are mostly used for the evaluation of the Fourier transform. Assume that f vanishes outside $[-K, K]$ and is sampled with stepsize h. Applying the trapezoidal rule to $\mathcal{F}(f)$ leads to the approximation

$$
\mathcal{F}(f)(\xi) = \frac{1}{\sqrt{2\pi}}h \sum_{n=-N}^{N-1} e^{-i\xi hn} f(hn) \, ,
$$

where $N = K/h$. Since $\mathcal{F}(f)$ is band-limited with bandwidth K, $\mathcal{F}(f)$ needs to be sampled with stepsize $\leq \pi/K$. If we choose the coarsest possible stepzise π/K, we have to evaluate

$$\mathcal{F}(f)(m\pi/K) = \frac{1}{\sqrt{2\pi}}h \sum_{n=-N}^{N-1} e^{-i\pi mn/N} f(hn) \qquad (2.12)$$

for $m = -N, \ldots, N-1$. Evaluating (2.12) is a discrete Fourier transform of length $2N$ and requires $O(N^2)$ complex multiplications and additions. Any algorithm of lower complexity, usually $O(N \log_2 N)$, is called a fast Fourier transform. The possibility of doing this arises from observing redundancies and reorganizing the calculations. Standard references are [106, 31]. We briefly describe the well-known FFT algorithm of Cooley and Tukey for N a power of 2. The basic idea in the Cooley-Tukey algorithm is to break the sum into one part with n even and the rest with n odd. We have

$$\mathcal{F}(f)(2m\pi/K) = \frac{1}{\sqrt{2\pi}}h \sum_{n=-N/2}^{N/2-1} e^{\frac{-i\pi mn}{N/2}} (f(hn) + f(h(n+N/2))) ,$$

and

$$\mathcal{F}(f)((2m+1)\pi/K) = \frac{1}{\sqrt{2\pi}}h \sum_{n=-N/2}^{N/2-1} e^{\frac{-i\pi mn}{N/2}} (f(hn) - f(h(n+N/2))) .$$

A discrete Fourier transform of length $2N$ may thus be calculated with two discrete Fourier transforms of size N plus $O(N)$ operations. If this is done in a recursive way we arrive at $C(N) = O(N \log_2 N)$, where $C(N)$ is the number of elementary operations needed to compute a discrete Fourier transform with the FFT. In fact, we have $C(N) = 2C(N/2) + O(N)$. With the change of variable $l = \log_2 N$ and the change of function $T(l) = C(N)/N$, we derive that $T(l) = T(l-1) + O(1)$. Since $C(1) = 0$ we obtain $T(l) = O(l)$ and in turn $C(N) = O(N \log_2 N)$.

2.4 The Two-Dimensional Radon Transform

Let θ be on the unit circle S^1, and take $p \in \mathbb{R}$. The equation $x \cdot \theta = p$ represents the line L which has (signed) distance p from origin and is perpendicular to the direction θ.

For any continuous function f of compact support, we can compute the line integral, with respect to Euclidean arc length ds,

$$Rf(\theta, p) := \int_{x \cdot \theta = p} f(x) \, ds = \int_{-\infty}^{+\infty} f(x_0 + t\theta^\perp) \, dt ,$$

where x_0 is a fixed point on L and $\theta^\perp$ is the rotate of θ by $\pi/2$.

The map $f \mapsto Rf$ is called the Radon transform and Rf is called the Radon transform of f. Clearly Rf is a function defined on $S^1 \times \mathbb{R}$ with the compatibility condition: $Rf(-\theta, -p) = Rf(\theta, p)$.

There are several reasonable domains of definition for R such as $L^1(\mathbb{R}^2)$ and $\mathcal{S}(\mathbb{R}^2)$, but in many applications it is enough to consider functions which are of compact support, with singularities which are only jumps along reasonable curves, and otherwise smooth.

Some easy properties of the Radon transform are obtained by observing that Rf can be written using distributions. In fact, if we introduce the unit density $\delta_{p-x\cdot\theta}$ which is supported by the line $x \cdot \theta = p$, then

$$Rf(\theta, p) = \int_{\mathbb{R}^2} f(x)\delta_{p-x\cdot\theta}\, dx , \qquad (2.13)$$

with the usual abuse of language.

It is also convenient to write

$$R_\theta(f) = Rf(\theta, p) .$$

Using the fact that $\delta_{p-x\cdot\theta}$ is homogeneous of degree -1, Rf can be extended to $\mathbb{R}^2 \setminus \{0\} \times \mathbb{R}$ as follows

$$Rf(\xi, s) = \frac{1}{|\xi|} Rf(\frac{\xi}{|\xi|}, \frac{s}{|\xi|}) .$$

We can therefore take derivatives of (2.13) with respect to the variables $\xi_j (\xi = (\xi_1, \xi_2))$ and obtain

$$\frac{\partial}{\partial \xi_j} Rf(\xi, s) = \int_{\mathbb{R}^2} f(x)\frac{\partial}{\partial \xi_j}\delta_{s-x\cdot\xi}\, dx, \quad j = 1, 2 ,$$

but

$$\frac{\partial}{\partial \xi_j}\delta_{s-x\cdot\xi} = -x_j\delta'_{s-x\cdot\xi} ,$$

and

$$\frac{\partial}{\partial s}\delta_{s-x\cdot\xi} = \delta'_{s-x\cdot\xi} ,$$

so that

$$\frac{\partial}{\partial \xi_j} Rf(\xi, s) = -\int_{\mathbb{R}^2} f(x)x_j\delta'_{s-x\cdot\xi}\, dx$$

$$= -\frac{\partial}{\partial s}\int_{\mathbb{R}^2} f(x)x_j\delta_{s-x\cdot\xi}\, dx$$

$$= -\frac{\partial}{\partial s}\Big[R(x_jf)(\xi, s)\Big].$$

On the other hand the Radon transform of the derivative of f is

$$R_\xi(\frac{\partial f}{\partial x_j})(s) = \int_{\mathbb{R}^2} \frac{\partial f}{\partial x_j}(x)\delta_{s-x\cdot\xi}\, dx$$

$$= \xi_j \int_{\mathbb{R}^2} f(x)\delta'_{s-x\cdot\xi}\, dx$$

$$= \xi_j \frac{\partial}{\partial s}(R_\xi f)(s) .$$

In particular, we obtain

$$R_\xi(\Delta f)(s) = (\xi_1^2 + \xi_2^2)\frac{\partial^2}{\partial s^2}(R_\xi f)(s) \ .$$

In other words, the Radon transform intertwines Δ and $\partial^2/\partial s^2$ when the arguments are restricted to $S^1 \times \mathbb{R}$.

Another useful property is the following.

Lemma 2.4.1 *Let $f, g \in \mathcal{S}(\mathbb{R}^2)$. Then*

$$R_\theta(f \star g) = R_\theta(f) \star R_\theta(g) \ . \tag{2.14}$$

The easiest way to verify (2.14) is via the Fourier Slice theorem, which we recall here.

Theorem 2.4.2 (Fourier Slice Theorem) *Let $f \in \mathcal{S}(\mathbb{R}^2)$. Then for $\theta \in S^1, s \in \mathbb{R}$,*

$$\mathcal{F}(R_\theta f)(s) = \sqrt{2\pi}\mathcal{F}(f)(s\theta) \ .$$

Proof. The proof is as follows,

$$\begin{aligned}
\mathcal{F}(R_\theta f)(s) &= \frac{1}{\sqrt{2\pi}} \int_{-\infty}^{+\infty} e^{-its} R_\theta(f)(t)\, dt \\
&= \frac{1}{\sqrt{2\pi}} \int_{-\infty}^{+\infty} e^{-its} \left[\int_{-\infty}^{+\infty} f(t\theta + s\theta^\perp)\, ds \right] dt \\
&= \frac{1}{\sqrt{2\pi}} \int_{\mathbb{R}^2} e^{-its} f(t\theta + s\theta^\perp)\, ds\, dt \ .
\end{aligned}$$

Letting now $x = t\theta + s\theta^\perp$, we have $t = x \cdot \theta$ and $dt\, ds = dx$, the Lebesgue measure in $\mathbb{R}^2$. Therefore,

$$\mathcal{F}(R_\theta f)(s) = \frac{1}{\sqrt{2\pi}} \int_{\mathbb{R}^2} e^{-isx\cdot\theta} f(x)\, dx = \sqrt{2\pi}\mathcal{F}(f)(s\theta) \ .$$

$\square$

Recalling now that in $\mathbb{R}^2$

$$\mathcal{F}(f \star g) = 2\pi\mathcal{F}(f)\mathcal{F}(g) \ ,$$

we can easily prove (2.14).

Let us also note that if τ_a denotes the translation by a, *i.e.*, $\tau_a f(x) = f(x - a)$, then

$$R(\tau_a f)(\theta, p) = R_\theta f(p - \theta \cdot a) = \tau_{\theta\cdot a} R_\theta f(p) \ .$$

2.5 The Moore-Penrose Generalized Inverse

Let A be a bounded operator from a Hilbert space H into a Hilbert space K. Let A^* denote the adjoint of A (see for example [118, page 487]). The Moore-Penrose generalized solution f^+ to $Af = g$ is defined as follows: f^+ is the element with the smallest norm in the set of the minimizers of $\|Af - g\|$ (if this set is nonempty, i.e., if $g \in \text{Range}(A) + \text{Range}(A)^\perp$). It can be shown that f^+ is the unique solution to the normal equation

$$A^*Af = A^*g$$

in $\overline{\text{Range}(A^*)}$. The linear operator A^+ defined by

$$f^+ = A^+g \quad \text{for } g \in \text{Range}(A) + \text{Range}(A)^\perp$$

is called the Moore-Penrose generalized inverse.

2.6 Singular Value Decomposition

Let A be a bounded linear operator from a Hilbert space H into a Hilbert space K. By the singular value decomposition (SVD) we mean a representation of A in the form

$$Af = \sum_l \sigma_l \left(f, f_l\right) g_l \ ,$$

where $(f_l), (g_l)$ are orthonormal systems in H, K, respectively, and σ_l are positive numbers, the singular values of A. The sum may be finite or infinite. The adjoint of A is given by

$$A^*g = \sum_l \sigma_l \left(g, g_l\right) f_l \ ,$$

and the operators

$$A^*Af = \sum_l \sigma_l^2 \left(f, f_l\right) f_l \ ,$$

$$AA^*g = \sum_l \sigma_l^2 \left(g, g_l\right) g_l \ ,$$

are self-adjoint operators in H, K, respectively. The spectrum of A^*A, AA^* consists of the eigenvalues σ_l^2 and possibly the eigenvalue 0, whose multiplicity may be infinite.

The Moore-Penrose generalized inverse is given by

$$A^+g = \sum_l \sigma_l^{-1} \left(g, g_l\right) f_l \ .$$

Let us now review the basic concepts of singular value decomposition of a matrix. Let $M_{m,n}(\mathbb{C})$ denote the set of all m-by-n matrices over $\mathbb{C}$.

The set $M_{n,n}(\mathbb{C})$ is abbreviated to $M_n(\mathbb{C})$. The spectral theorem applied to the positive semi-definite matrices AA^* and A^*A gives the following singular value decomposition of a matrix $A \in M_{m,n}(\mathbb{C})$. Here $A^* := \overline{A}^T$, where T denotes the transpose.

Theorem 2.6.1 (Spectral Theorem) *Let $A \in M_{m,n}(\mathbb{C})$ be given, and let $q = \min\{m,n\}$. There is a matrix $\Sigma = (\Sigma_{ij}) \in M_{m,n}(\mathbb{R})$ with $\Sigma_{ij} = 0$ for all $i \neq j$ and $\Sigma_{11} \geq \Sigma_{22} \geq \ldots \geq \Sigma_{qq} \geq 0$, and there are two unitary matrices $V \in M_m(\mathbb{C})$ and $W \in M_n(\mathbb{C})$ such that $A = V\Sigma W^*$. The numbers $\{\Sigma_{ii}\}$ are the nonnegative square roots of the eigenvalues of AA^*, and hence are uniquely determined. The columns of V are eigenvectors of AA^* and the columns of W are eigenvectors of A^*A (arranged in the same order as the corresponding eigenvalues Σ_{ii}^2).*

The diagonal entries Σ_{ii}, $i = 1, \ldots, q = \min\{m,n\}$ of Σ are called the singular values of A, and the columns of V and the columns of W are the (respectively, left and right) singular vectors of A.

SVD has the following desirable computational properties:

(i) The rank of A can be easily determined from its SVD. Specifically, rank(A) equals to the number of nonzero singular values of A.
(ii) The L_2-norm of A is given by $\|A\|_2 = \sqrt{\sum_{m=1}^{q} \Sigma_{mm}^2}$.
(iii) SVD is an effective computational tool for finding lower-rank approximations to a given matrix. Specifically, let $p < \text{rank}(A)$. Then the rank p matrix A_p minimizing $\|A - A_p\|_2$ is given by $A_p = V\Sigma_p W^*$, where the matrix Σ_p is obtained from Σ after the singular values $\Sigma_{nn}, p+1 \leq n \leq q$, are set to zero.

2.7 Compact Operators

Let H be a Banach space. A bounded linear operator A is compact if whenever $\{x_j\}$ is a bounded sequence in H, the sequence $\{Ax_j\}$ has a convergent subsequence. The operator A is said to be of finite rank if Range(A) is finite-dimensional. Clearly every operator of finite rank is compact.

We recall some basic results on compact operators.

(i) The set of compact operators on H is a closed two-sided ideal in the algebra of bounded operators on H with the norm topology.
(ii) If A is a bounded operator on the Banach space H and there is a sequence $\{A_N\}_{N \in \mathbb{N}}$ of operators of finite rank such that $\|A_N - A\| \to 0$, then A is compact.
(iii) The operator A is compact on the Banach space H if and only if the dual operator A^* is compact on the dual space H^*.

We also recall the main structure theorem for compact operators. Let A be a compact operator on the Hilbert space H (which we identify with its dual).

For each $\lambda \in \mathbb{C}$, let $V_\lambda = \{x \in X : Ax = \lambda x\}$ and $V_{\overline{\lambda}} = \{x \in X : A^*x = \overline{\lambda}x\}$. Then

(i) The set of $\lambda \in \mathbb{C}$ for which $V_\lambda \neq \{0\}$ is finite or countable, and in the latter case its only accumulation point is zero. Moreover, $\dim(V_\lambda) < +\infty$ for all $\lambda \neq 0$.
(ii) If $\lambda \neq 0, \dim(V_\lambda) = \dim(V_{\overline{\lambda}})$.
(iii) If $\lambda \neq 0$, the range of $\lambda I - A$ is closed.

Suppose $\lambda \neq 0$. Then

(i) The equation $(\lambda I - A)x = y$ has a solution if and only if $y \perp V_{\overline{\lambda}}$.
(ii) $(\lambda I - A)$ is surjective if and only if it is injective.

We recall the concept of a Fredholm operator acting between Banach spaces H and K. We say that a bounded linear operator $A : H \to K$ is Fredholm if the subspace $\text{Range}(A)$ is closed in K and the subspaces $\text{Ker}(A)$ and $K/\text{Range}(A)$ are finite-dimensional. In this case, the index of A is the integer defined by

$$\text{index }(A) = \dim \text{Ker}(A) - \dim(K/\text{Range}(A)) .$$

In the sequel, we encapsulate the main conclusion of Fredholm's original theory. If $A = I + B$, where $B : H \to H$ is compact, then $A : H \to H$ is Fredholm with index zero. This shows that the index is stable under compact perturbations. If $A : H \to K$ is Fredholm and $B : H \to K$ is compact, then their sum $A + B : H \to K$ is Fredholm, and $\text{index }(A + B) = \text{index }(A)$.

2.8 Regularization of Ill-Posed Problems

In this section we review some of the most commonly used methods for solving ill-posed inverse problems. These methods are called regularization methods. Although the emphasis in this book is not on classical regularization techniques, it is quite important to understand the philosophy behind them and how they work in practice.

2.8.1 Stability

Problems in image reconstruction are usually not well-posed in the sense of Hadamard. This means that they suffer from one of the following deficiencies:

(i) They are not solvable (in the strict sense) at all.
(ii) They are not uniquely solvable.
(iii) The solution does not depend continuously on the data.

To explain the basic ideas of regularization, let A be a bounded linear operator from a Hilbert space H into a Hilbert space K. Consider the problem of solving

$$Af = g \qquad (2.15)$$

for f.(i) means that g is not in the range of A, (ii) means that A is not injective, and (iii) means that A^{-1} is not continuous.

One could do away with (i) and (ii) by using the generalized inverse A^+. But A^+ does not have to be continuous. Thus, small error in g may cause errors of arbitrary size in f. To restore continuity, we introduce the notion of a regularization of A^+. This is a family $(T_\gamma)_{\gamma>0}$ of linear continuous operators $T_\gamma : K \to H$, which are defined on all of K and for which

$$\lim_{\gamma \to 0} T_\gamma g = A^+ g$$

on the domain of A^+. Obviously, $||T_\gamma|| \to +\infty$ as $\gamma \to 0$ if A^+ is unbounded. With the help of regularization, we can solve (2.15) in the following way. Let $g^\epsilon \in K$ be an approximation to g such that $||g - g^\epsilon|| \leq \epsilon$. Let $\gamma(\epsilon)$ be such that, as $\epsilon \to 0$,

$$\gamma(\epsilon) \to 0, \quad ||T_{\gamma(\epsilon)}|| \, \epsilon \to 0 \; .$$

Then, as $\epsilon \to 0$,

$$
\begin{aligned}
||T_{\gamma(\epsilon)} g^\epsilon - A^+ g|| &\leq ||T_{\gamma(\epsilon)}(g^\epsilon - g)|| + ||T_{\gamma(\epsilon)} g - A^+ g|| \\
&\leq ||T_{\gamma(\epsilon)}|| \, \epsilon + ||T_{\gamma(\epsilon)} g - A^+ g|| \\
&\to 0 \; .
\end{aligned}
$$

Hence $T_{\gamma(\epsilon)} g^\epsilon$ is close to $A^+ g$ if g^ϵ is close to g.

The number γ is called a regularization parameter. Determining a good regularization parameter is a major issue in the theory of ill-posed problems.

A classical ill-posed inverse problem is the deconvolution problem. Define the compact operator $A : L^2(\mathbb{R}) \to L^2(\mathbb{R})$ by

$$(Af)(x) := \int_{-\infty}^{+\infty} h(x - y) f(y) \, dy \; ,$$

where h is a Gaussian convolution kernel,

$$h(x) := \frac{1}{\sqrt{2\pi}} e^{-x^2/2} \; .$$

The operator A is injective, which can be seen by applying the Fourier transform on Af, yielding

$$\mathcal{F}(Af) = \mathcal{F}(h \star f) = \mathcal{F}(h)\mathcal{F}(f) \; ,$$

with $\mathcal{F}(h)$ given by (2.8). Therefore, if $Af = 0$, we have $\mathcal{F}(f) = 0$, hence $f = 0$. Formally, the solution to the equation $Af = g$ is

$$f(x) = \mathcal{F}^{-1}\left(\frac{\mathcal{F}(g)}{\mathcal{F}(h)}\right)(x), \quad x \in \mathbb{R} . \tag{2.16}$$

However, the above formula is not well defined for general $g \in L^2(\mathbb{R})$ (or even in $\mathcal{S}'(\mathbb{R})$) since $1/\mathcal{F}(h)$ grows exponentially.

Measurement errors of arbitrarily small L^2-norm in g may cause g to be not in Range(A) and the inversion formula (2.16) practically useless.

The basic idea of regularization is that, instead of trying to solve (2.15) exactly, one seeks to find a nearby problem that is uniquely solvable and that is robust in the sense that small errors in the data do not corrupt excessively this approximate solution.

We briefly discuss three families of classical regularization methods: (i) regularization by singular value truncation, (ii) the Tikhonov-Phillips regularization and (iii) regularization by truncated iterative methods.

2.8.2 The Truncated SVD

Let

$$Af = \sum_l \sigma_l \, (f, f_l) \, g_l$$

be the SVD of A. Then

$$T_\gamma g = \sum_{\sigma_l \geq \gamma} \sigma_l^{-1} \, (g, g_l) \, f_l \tag{2.17}$$

is a regularization with $\|T_\gamma\| \leq 1/\gamma$.

A good measure for the degree of ill-posedness of (2.15) is the rate of decay of the singular value σ_l. It is clear from (2.17) that the ill-posedness is more pronounced as the rate of decay increases. A polynomial decay is usually considered manageable, while an exponential decay indicates that only very poor approximations to f in (2.15) can be computed. The SVD gives us all the information we need about an ill-posed problem.

There is a rule for choosing the truncation level, that is often referred to as the discrepancy principle. This principle states that we cannot expect the approximate solution to yield a smaller residual error, $Af_\gamma - g$, than the noise level ϵ, since otherwise we would be fitting the solution to the noise. It leads to the following selection criterion for γ: choose the largest γ that satisfies $\|g - \sum_{\sigma_l \geq \gamma}(g, g_l)g_l\| \leq \epsilon$.

2.8.3 Tikhonov-Phillips Regularization

Linear Problems

The discussion in the above subsection demonstrates that when solving the equation (2.15) for a compact operator A, serious problems occur when the singular values of A tend to zero rapidly, causing the norm of the approximate solution to go to infinity as the regularization parameter γ goes to zero. The idea in the basic Tikhonov-Phillips regularization scheme is to control simultaneously the norm of the residual, $Af_\gamma - g$, and the norm of the approximate solution f_γ.

To do so, we set

$$T_\gamma = (A^*A + \gamma I)^{-1} A^* .$$

Equivalently, $f_\gamma = T_\gamma g$ can be defined by minimizing $||Af - g||^2 + \gamma ||f||^2$. Here the regularization parameter γ plays essentially the role of a Lagrange multiplier. In terms of the SVD of A, we have

$$T_\gamma g = \sum_l F_\gamma(\sigma_l)\sigma_l^{-1} (g, g_l) f_l ,$$

where $F_\gamma(\sigma) = \sigma^2/(\sigma^2 + \gamma)$.

The choice of the value of the regularization parameter γ based on the noise level of the measurement g is a central issue in the literature discussing Tikhonov-Phillips regularization. Several methods for choosing γ have been proposed. The most common one is known as the Morozov discrepancy principle. This principle is essentially the same as the discrepancy principle discussed in connection with the singular value truncation principle. It is rather straightforward to implement numerically.

Let ϵ be the measurement error. Let

$$\varphi : \mathbb{R}^+ \to \mathbb{R}^+, \quad \varphi(\gamma) = ||Af_\gamma - g||$$

be the discrepancy related to the regularization parameter γ. The Morozov discrepancy principle says that γ should be chosen from the condition

$$f(\gamma) = \epsilon , \tag{2.18}$$

if possible, *i.e.*, the regularized solution should not try to satisfy the data more accurately than up to the noise level. Equation (2.18) has a unique solution $\gamma = \gamma(\epsilon)$ if and only if (i) any component in the data g that is orthogonal to Range(A) must be due to noise and (ii) the error level should not exceed the signal level.

Nonlinear Problems

Tikhonov-Phillips regularization method is sometimes applicable also when non-linear problems are considered. Let H_1 and H_2 be (real) Hilbert spaces. Let $A : H_1 \to H_2$ be a nonlinear mapping. We want to find $f \in H_1$ satisfying

$$A(f) = g + \epsilon , \tag{2.19}$$

where ϵ is observation noise. If A is such that large changes in f may produce small changes in $A(f)$, the problem of finding f solution to (2.19) is ill-posed and numerical methods, typically, iterative ones, may fail to find a satisfactory estimate of f.

The nonlinear Tikhonov-Phillips regularization scheme amounts to searching for f that minimizes the functional

$$||A(f) - g||^2 + \gamma G(f) , \qquad (2.20)$$

where $G : H_1 \to \mathbb{R}$ is a nonnegative functional. The most common penalty term is $G(f) = ||f||^2$. We restrict ourselves to this choice and suppose that A is Fréchet differentiable. In this case, the most common method to search for a minimizer of (2.20) is to use an iterative scheme based on successive linearizations of A. The linearization of A around a given point f_0 leads that the minimizer of (2.20) (around f_0) is

$$f = (R_{f_0}^* R_{f_0} + \gamma I)^{-1} R_{f_0}^* \left(g - A(f_0) + R_{f_0} f_0 \right),$$

where R_{f_0} is the Fréchet derivative of A at f_0. We recall that A is Fréchet differentiable at f_0 if it allows an expansion of the form

$$A(f_0 + h) = A(f_0) + R_{f_0} h + o(||h||) ,$$

where R_{f_0} is a continuous linear operator.

2.8.4 Regularization by Truncated Iterative Methods

The most common iterative methods are Landweber iteration, Kaczmarz iteration, and Krylov subspace methods. The best known of the Krylov iterative methods when the matrix A is symmetric and positive definite is the conjugate gradient method. In this section, we only discuss regularizing properties of Landweber and Kaczmarz iterations. We refer to [74] and the references therein concerning the Krylov subspace methods.

Landweber Iteration

The drawback of the Thikhonov-Phillips regularization is that it requires to invert the regularization of the normal operator $A^* A + \gamma I$. This inversion may be costly in practice. The Landweber iteration method is an iterative technique in which no inversion is necessary. It is defined to solve the equation $Af = g$ as follows

$$f^0 = 0, \quad f^{k+1} = (I - rA^*A)f^k + rA^*g, \quad k \geq 0 ,$$

for some $r > 0$. By induction, we verify that $f^k = T_\gamma g$, with $\gamma = 1/k, k \geq 1$, and

$$T_\gamma = r \sum_{l=0}^{1/\gamma - 1} (I - rA^*A)^l A^* = \sum_{l=1}^{+\infty} \frac{1}{\sigma_l}(1 - (1 - r\sigma_l^2)^{1/\gamma})(g, g_l) f_l .$$

Kaczmarz Iteration

Kaczmarz's method is an iterative method for solving linear systems of equations. Let $H, H_j, j = 1, \ldots, p$, be (real) Hilbert spaces, and let

$$A_j : H \to H_j, \quad j = 1, \ldots, p,$$

be linear continuous maps from H onto H_j. Let $g_j \in H_j$ be given. We want to compute $f \in H$ such that

$$A_j f = g_j, \quad j = 1, \ldots, p. \tag{2.21}$$

Kaczmarz's method for the solution of (2.21) reads:

$$f_0 = f^k,$$
$$f_j = f_{j-1} + \gamma A_j^* (A_j A_j^*)^{-1} (g_j - A_j f_{j-1}), \quad j = 1, \ldots, p,$$
$$f^{k+1} = f_p,$$

with $f^0 \in H$ arbitrary. Here γ is a regularization parameter. Under certain assumptions, f^k converges to a solution of (2.21) if (2.21) has a solution and to a generalized solution if not.

2.9 General Image Characteristics

Irrespective to the method used to acquire medical images, there are a number of criteria by which the image characteristics can be evaluated and compared. The most important of these criteria are spatial resolution and the signal-to-noise ratio. This section covers a number of general concepts applicable to all the imaging modalities in this book.

2.9.1 Spatial Resolution

There are a number of measures used to describe the spatial resolution of an imaging modality. We focus on describing a point spread function (PSF) concept and show how to use it to analyze resolution limitation in several practical imaging schemes.

Point Spread Function

Consider an idealized object consisting of a single point. It is likely that the image we obtain from it is a blurred point. Nevertheless, we are still able to identify it as a point. Now, we add another point to the object. If the two points are farther apart, we will see two blurred points. However, as the two points are moving closer to each other, the image looks less two points. In fact, the two points will merge together to become a single blob when their separation is below a certain threshold. We call this threshold value the resolution limit of the imaging system. Formally stated, the spatial resolution of an imaging system is the smallest separation of two point sources necessary for them to remain resolvable in the resultant image. In order to arrive at a more quantitative definition of the resolution, we next introduce the point spread function concept. The relationship between an arbitrary object function $I(x)$ and its image $\hat{I}$ is described by $\hat{I}(x) = I(x) * h(x)$, where the convolution kernel function $h(x)$ is known as the point spread function since $\hat{I}(x) = h(x)$ for $I(x) = \delta_x$. In a perfect imaging system, the PSF $h(x)$ would be a delta function, and in this case the image would be a perfect representation of the object. If $h(x)$ deviates from a δ−function, $\hat{I}(x)$ will be a blurred version of $I(x)$. The amount of blurring introduced to $\hat{I}(x)$ by an imperfect $h(x)$ can be quantified by the width of $h(x)$. The spatial resolution, W_h, is clearly related to the PSF. It is defined as the full width of $h(x)$ at its half maximum.

If the PSF is a sinc function,

$$h(x) = \frac{\sin kx}{kx}(= j_0(kx)) ,$$

then this definition of resolution coincides with the Rayleigh criterion which states that the two point sources can be resolved if the peak intensity of the *sinc* PSF from one source coincides with the first zero-crossing point of the PSF of the other, *i.e.*, if the two source points are separated by one-half the wavelength $\lambda := 2\pi/k$. If the PSF is given by

$$h(x) = \frac{J_1(kx)}{kx} ,$$

J_1 being the Bessel function of the first order, then the Rayleigh resolution limit is given by $W_h \approx 0.61\lambda$ since the first zero of J_1 is approximately 3.83.

If the PSF is a Gaussian function,

$$h(x) = \frac{1}{\sqrt{2\pi\sigma^2}}e^{-(x-x_0)^2/\sigma^2} ,$$

where σ is the deviation of the distribution and x_0 is the center of the function, then the resolution is given by $2\sqrt{2\ln 2}\sigma \approx 2.36\,\sigma$.

Consider now the problem of reconstructing an image from its truncated Fourier series. The image reconstructed based on the truncated Fourier series is given by

$$\hat{I}(x) = \frac{1}{\sqrt{2\pi}}\Delta k \sum_{n=-N/2}^{N/2-1} S(n\Delta k)e^{in\Delta k\,x} ,$$

where $S(n\Delta k) = \frac{1}{\sqrt{2\pi}}\int_{\mathbb{R}} I(x)e^{-in\Delta k\,x}\,dx$. The underlying PSF is given by

$$h(x) = \Delta k\,\frac{\sin(\pi N\Delta k\,x)}{\sin(\pi\Delta k\,x)} ,$$

with Δk being the fundamental frequency and N the number of Fourier samples. Then the full width of h at its half maximum is $W_h = 1/(N\Delta k)$. Therefore, we cannot improve image resolution and reduce the number of measured data points at the same time. This assertion is often referred to as the uncertainty relation of Fourier imaging, and in practice, one chooses N as large as signal-to-noise ratio and imaging time permit.

2.9.2 Signal-To-Noise Ratio

Imaging involves measurement and processing of activated signals from an object. Any practical measurement always contains an undesirable component that is uncorrelated with the desired signal. This component is referred to as noise or a random signal. Of great concern to imaging scientists is the question of how noise is picked up or generated in an imaging system and how the imaging process handles it-that is, whether it is suppressed or amplified. The first aspect of the topic is related mostly to the imaging system hardware and will not be discussed here. The second aspect is related to the mathematical and processing principles used for the image formation and is discussed in this section. We begin with a review of some fundamental concepts of noise signals.

Random Variables

A characteristic of noise is that it does not have fixed values in repeated measurements. Such a quantity is described by a random variable and follows a certain statistical relationship, known as the probability density function (PDF). The PDF of a random variable ξ is often denoted as $p_\xi(x)$, which represents the probability of obtaining a specific value x for ξ in a particular measurement, the area under any PDF must be one. The mean of a random variable, ξ, is defined as

$$E[\xi] = \int x p_\xi(x)\, dx \ .$$

It is the first-order statistical moment. The variance is defined as

$$\mathrm{var}[\xi] = E[|\xi - E[\xi]|^2] \ ,$$

which is a second-order statistical moment. $\sigma_\xi := \sqrt{\mathrm{var}[\xi]}$ is called the standard deviation, which is a measure of the average deviation from the mean.

The PDF of measurement noise is not always known in practical situations. We often use parameters such as mean and variance to describe it. In fact, based on the central limit theorem, most measurement noise can be treated as Gaussian noise, in which case the PDF is uniquely defined by its mean and variance. Recall here the central limit theorem: When a function $h(x)$ is convolved with itself n times, in the limit $n \to +\infty$, the convolution product is a Gaussian function with a variance that is n times the variance of $h(x)$, provided the area, mean, and variance of $h(x)$ are finite. This theorem can be interpreted as saying that convolution is a smoothing process. Therefore, it is often appropriate to say that an image obtained from a practical imaging system is a smooth version of the true image (or object) function.

The PDF of a Gaussian random variable is

$$p_\xi(x) = \frac{1}{\sqrt{2\pi}\sigma} e^{-(x-x_0)^2/2\sigma^2} .$$

It can be shown that $E[\xi] = x_0$ and $\mathrm{var}[\xi] = \sigma^2$.

Let $\hat{I} = I + \xi$ be a measured quantity containing the true signal I and the noise component ξ with zero mean and standard deviation σ_ξ. The signal-to-noise ratio (SNR) for $\hat{I}$ from a single measurement is defined by

$$(S/N)_{\hat{I}} = \frac{|I|}{\sigma_\xi} .$$

If N measurements are taken such that $\hat{I}_n = I + \xi_n$ are obtained to produce

$$\frac{1}{N} \sum_{n=1}^{N} \hat{I}_n = I + \frac{1}{N} \sum_{n=1}^{N} \xi_n ,$$

then the signal-to-noise ratio for $(1/N) \sum_{n=1}^{N} \hat{I}_n$ is

$$\frac{|I|}{\sqrt{\mathrm{var}[\frac{1}{N} \sum_{n=1}^{N} \xi_n]}} = \sqrt{N}\frac{|I|}{\sigma_\xi} = \sqrt{N}(S/N)_{\hat{I}} ,$$

assuming that the noise for different measurements is uncorrelated. Thus N signal averaging yields an improvement by a factor of $\sqrt{N}$ in the signal-to-noise ratio. Recall that two signals, ξ_1 and ξ_2, are said to be uncorrelated if

$$E[(\xi_1 - E[\xi_1])\overline{(\xi_2 - E[\xi_2])}] = 0.$$

Random Signals

Random signals picked up in an imaging experiment are described by functions with random values, which are known as random (or stochastic) processes. Denoting $\xi(t)$ as a random process, $\xi(t_0)$ for any time instant t_0 is a random variable, but each sample of $\xi(t)$ is a deterministic function of time. As in the case of random variables, we may not always require a complete statistical description of a random process, or we may not be able to obtain it even if desired. In such cases, we work with various statistical moments. The most important ones are

(i) Mean: $E[\xi(t)]$;

(ii) Variance: $\operatorname{var}[\xi(t)] = E[|\xi(t) - E[\xi(t)]|^2]$;

(iii) and the correlation function: $R(t, t + \tau) = E[\xi(t)\overline{\xi(t + \tau)}]$.

For some random processes, the mean and the variance are independent of time and the correlation function depends only on the time difference τ. Those processes are termed stationary. Another important property of random processes is ergodicity, which means that time and ensemble averages are interchangeable. For example, if $\xi(t)$ is an ergodic process, then

(i) $E[\xi(t)] = <\xi(t)>$,

(ii) $\operatorname{var}[\xi(t)] = <|\xi(t) - E[\xi(t)]|^2>$,

(iii) $R(\tau) := E[\xi(t)\overline{\xi(t + \tau)}] = <\xi(t)\overline{\xi(t + \tau)}>$,

where $< \cdot >$ is the time average operator, defined as

$$< \xi(t) > := \lim_{T \to +\infty} \frac{1}{2T} \int_{-T}^{T} \xi(t) \, dt .$$

Therefore, for ergodic processes, the statistical moments are measurable from any sample function. Furthermore, for an ergodic process, $R(\tau)$ is a deterministic function of time, and its Fourier transform gives the power spectral density function- a relationship established by the well-known Wiener theorem. If the spectral density function is a constant over the measurement frequency range, the noise is referred to as white noise in practice.

Noise signals we consider in this book are assumed to come from an ergodic, stationary, uncorrelated, white noise process.

Image Artifacts

Image distortion or artifacts often arise in tomographic imaging owing either to insufficient data or to inaccurate data, or both. An insufficiency of measured data occurs because of practical physical and temporal constraints in data acquisition. Data distortions are often due to imperfections in the data acquisition system. Gibbs ringing artifact and aliasing artifacts are very typical artifacts encountered in practice. Another typical artifact is motion artifact. Common motion artifacts are image blurring and ghost and are due to the object motion during the experiment. The interested reader is referred to [91, page 260] for a discussion on some concepts to understand motion effects and motion compensation techniques. Aliasing artifacts have been discussed in Sect. 2.3.1. Here, we only focus on Gibbs ringing artifact.

The Gibbs ringing artifact is a common image distortion that exists in Fourier images, which manifests itself as spurious ringing around sharp edges. It is a result of truncating the Fourier series model owing to finite sampling or missing of high-frequency data. It is fundamentally related to the convergence behavior of the Fourier series. Specifically, when $I(x)$ is a smooth function, $\hat{I}(x)$ given by

$$\hat{I}(x) = \frac{1}{\sqrt{2\pi}}\Delta k \sum_{n=-N/2}^{N/2-1} S(n\Delta k)e^{in\Delta k\,x} ,$$

uniformly converges to $I(x)$ as $N \to +\infty$ for bounded x. More precisely, if $I(x) \in C^p$, then $\|\hat{I}(x) - I(x)\|_2$ approaches zero on the order of $1/N^{p+1}$. If I has discontinuities then there is a nonuniform convergence of $\hat{I}$ to I in the vicinity of the discontinuous points of I. This nonuniform behavior of the limit $\hat{I}(x) \to I(x)$ as $N \to +\infty$ is called the Gibbs phenomenon.

An obvious way to reduce the Gibbs ringing artifact is to collect more high-frequency data. This may not be possible in practice because of practical physical or temporal constraints on data acquisition. Another approach is to filter the measured data before they are Fourier transformed. This operation is described by

$$\hat{I}(x) = \frac{1}{\sqrt{2\pi}}\Delta k \sum_{n=-N/2}^{N/2-1} S(n\Delta k)w_n e^{in\Delta k\,x} , \tag{2.22}$$

where w_n is a filter function. This method is motivated by the understanding that the Gibbs ringing artifact is directly related to the oscillatory nature of the PSF associated with rectangular window function implicitly used in the Fourier reconstruction method. With the reconstruction formula in (2.22), one can derive that the PSF is

$$h(x) = \frac{1}{\sqrt{2\pi}}\Delta k \sum_{n=-N/2}^{N/2-1} w_n e^{in\Delta k x} .$$

Therefore, by properly choosing the filter function w_n, one can significantly suppress the oscillations in $h(x)$, and thus the Gibbs ringing in $\hat{I}(x)$. A variety of filters have been proposed for this purpose. The most popular one is the Hamming filter defined by $w_n = H(2\pi n/N)$, where

$$H(x) := \begin{cases} 0.54 + 0.46\cos(2\pi x), & |x| \le 1/2 , \\ 0 & \text{otherwise.} \end{cases} \tag{2.23}$$

Although the filtering approach is effective in suppressing the Gibbs ringing, it is at the price of spatial resolution. This point can be understood by examining the effective width of the resulting PSF. Specifically,

$$W_h = \frac{1}{\Delta k \sum_{n=-N/2}^{N/2-1} w_n} \frac{\Delta k}{2\pi} \int_{-\frac{\pi}{\Delta k}}^{\frac{\pi}{\Delta k}} \sum_{n=-N/2}^{N/2-1} w_n e^{in\Delta k x}\, dx$$

$$= \frac{1}{\sum_{n=-N/2}^{N/2-1}(w_n/w_0)\Delta k} .$$

Since $w_n \ge w_0$ for any practical filter function used for this purpose, we have

$$W_h \geq \frac{1}{N \Delta k} \, .$$

This equation asserts that the filtering operation is a lossy process in terms of image resolution. To overcome this problem, various sophisticated reconstruction methods have been proposed. See [91].

Bibliography and Discussion

For reference books (written by mathematicians for mathematicians) on Radon transform we recommend [65, 96]. For a complete account of the mathematical theory of regularization of inverse problems, the reader is referred to the book by Engl, Hanke, and Neubauer [52]. See [74] where regularization methods are analyzed from the point of view of statics. A convergence proof of the Kaczmarz's method can be found in the book [102].

3

Layer Potential Techniques

The anomaly detection algorithms described in this book rely on asymptotic expansions of the fields when the medium contains anomalies of small volume. Such asymptotics will be investigated in the case of the conduction equation, the Helmholtz equation, the operator of elasticity, and the Stokes system. As it will be shown in the subsequent chapters, a remarkable feature of these imaging techniques, is that they allow a stable and accurate reconstruction of the location and of the geometric features of the anomalies, even for moderately noisy data.

We prepare the way in this chapter by reviewing a number of basic facts on the layer potentials for these equations which are very useful for anomaly detection. The most important results in this chapter are what we call decomposition theorems for transmission problems. For such problems, we prove that the solution is the sum of two functions, one solving the homogeneous problem, the other inheriting geometric properties of the anomaly. These results have many applications. They have been used to prove global uniqueness results for anomaly detection problems [75, 77]. In this book, we will use them to provide asymptotic expansions of the solution perturbations due to presence of small volume anomalies.

We begin with proving a decomposition formula of the steady-state voltage potential into a harmonic part and a refraction part. We then discuss the transmission problem for the Helmholtz equation, and proceed to establish a decomposition formula for the solution to this problem. Compared to the conductivity equation, the only new difficulty in establishing a decomposition theorem for the Helmholtz equation is that the equations inside and outside the anomaly are not the same. We should then consider two unknowns and solve a system of equations on the boundary of the anomaly instead of just one equation. After that, we turn to elliptic systems, namely, the Lamé and the Stokes systems. We investigate the transmission problems for these systems and derive decomposition theorems for the solutions to the transmission problems. Due to the vectorial aspect of the equations, our derivations are more complicate and our analysis is more delicate than in the scalar cases. We also note that when dealing with exterior problems for the Helmholtz equation or the dynamic elasticity, one should introduce a radiation condition, known as the Sommerfeld radiation condition, to select the physical solution to the problem.

3.1 The Laplace Equation

This section deals with the Laplace operator (or Laplacian) in $\mathbb{R}^d$, denoted by Δ. The Laplacian constitutes the simplest example of an elliptic partial differential equation. After deriving the fundamental solution for the Laplacian, we shall introduce the single- and double-layer potentials. We then provide the jump relations and mapping properties of these surface potentials. The final subsection investigates the transmission problem.

3.1.1 Fundamental Solution

To give a fundamental solution to the Laplacian in the general case of the dimension d, we denote by ω_d the area of the unit sphere in $\mathbb{R}^d$. Even though the following result is elementary we give its proof for the reader's convenience.

Lemma 3.1.1 *A fundamental solution to the Laplacian is given by*

$$
\Gamma(x) = \begin{cases} \dfrac{1}{2\pi} \ln |x| \,, & d = 2, \\[2mm] \dfrac{1}{(2-d)\omega_d} |x|^{2-d} \,, & d \geq 3. \end{cases}
\tag{3.1}
$$

Proof. The Laplacian is radially symmetric, so it is natural to seek Γ in the form $\Gamma(x) = w(r)$ where $r = |x|$. Since

$$
\Delta w = \frac{d^2 w}{d^2 r} + \frac{(d-1)}{r} \frac{dw}{dr} = \frac{1}{r^{d-1}} \frac{d}{dr} \left(r^{d-1} \frac{dw}{dr} \right),
$$

$\Delta \Gamma = 0$ in $\mathbb{R}^d \setminus \{0\}$ forces that w must satisfy

$$
\frac{1}{r^{d-1}} \frac{d}{dr} \left(r^{d-1} \frac{dw}{dr} \right) = 0 \quad \text{for } r > 0,
$$

and hence

$$
w(r) = \begin{cases} \dfrac{a_d}{(2-d)} \dfrac{1}{r^{d-2}} + b_d & \text{when } d \geq 3, \\[2mm] a_2 \ln r + b_2 & \text{when } d = 2, \end{cases}
$$

for some constants a_d and b_d. The choice of b_d is arbitrary, but a_d is fixed by the requirement that $\Delta \Gamma = \delta_0$ in $\mathbb{R}^d$, where δ_0 is the Dirac function at 0, or in other words

$$\int_{\mathbb{R}^d} \Gamma \Delta\phi = \phi(0) \quad \text{for } \phi \in \mathcal{C}_0^\infty(\mathbb{R}^d) . \tag{3.2}$$

Any test function $\phi \in \mathcal{C}_0^\infty(\mathbb{R}^d)$ has compact support, so we can apply Green's formula over the unbounded domain $\{x : |x| > \epsilon\}$ to arrive at

$$
\begin{aligned}
\int_{|x|>\epsilon} \Gamma(x)\Delta\phi(x)\,dx &= \int_{|x|=\epsilon} \phi(x)\frac{\partial\Gamma}{\partial\nu}(x)\,d\sigma(x) \\
&\quad - \int_{|x|=\epsilon} \Gamma(x)\frac{\partial\phi}{\partial\nu}(x)\,d\sigma(x) ,
\end{aligned}
\tag{3.3}
$$

where $\nu = x/|x|$ on $\{|x| = \epsilon\}$. Since

$$\nabla\Gamma(x) = \frac{dw}{dr}\frac{x}{|x|} = \frac{a_d x}{|x|^d} \quad \text{for } d \geq 2 ,$$

we have

$$\frac{\partial\Gamma}{\partial\nu}(x) = a_d\epsilon^{1-d} \quad \text{for } |x| = \epsilon .$$

Thus by the continuity of ϕ,

$$\int_{|x|=\epsilon} \phi(x)\frac{\partial\Gamma}{\partial\nu}(x)\,d\sigma(x) = \frac{a_d}{\epsilon^{d-1}} \int_{|x|=\epsilon} \phi(x)\,d\sigma(x) \to a_d\omega_d\phi(0)$$

as $\epsilon \to 0$, whereas

$$\int_{|x|=\epsilon} \Gamma(x)\frac{\partial\phi}{\partial\nu}(x)\,d\sigma(x) = \begin{cases} O(\epsilon) & \text{if } d \geq 3 , \\ O(\epsilon|\ln\epsilon|) & \text{if } d = 2 . \end{cases}$$

Thus, if $a_d = 1/\omega_d$, then (3.2) follows from (3.3) after sending $\epsilon \to 0$. $\square$

Let $p \in \mathbb{R}^d$ and $q \in \mathbb{R}$. The function $q\Gamma(x-z)$ is called the potential due to charges q at the source point z. The function $p \cdot \nabla_z \Gamma(x-z)$ is called the dipole of moment $|p|$ and direction $p/|p|$. It is known that using point charges one can realize a dipole only approximately (two large charges a small distance apart). See [108].

Now we prove Green's identity.

Lemma 3.1.2 *Assume that D is a bounded $\mathcal{C}^2$-domain in $\mathbb{R}^d, d \geq 2$, and let $u \in W^{1,2}(D)$ be a harmonic function. Then for any $x \in D$,*

$$u(x) = \int_{\partial D} \left(u(y)\frac{\partial\Gamma}{\partial\nu_y}(x-y) - \frac{\partial u}{\partial\nu_y}(y)\Gamma(x-y) \right) d\sigma(y) . \tag{3.4}$$

Proof. For $x \in D$ let $B_\epsilon(x)$ be the ball of center x and radius ϵ. We apply Green's formula to u and $\Gamma(x - \cdot)$ in the domain $D \setminus \overline{B_\epsilon}$ for small ϵ and get

$$\int_{D \setminus B_\epsilon(x)} \left(\Gamma \Delta u - u \Delta \Gamma \right) dy = \int_{\partial D} \left(\Gamma \frac{\partial u}{\partial \nu} - u \frac{\partial \Gamma}{\partial \nu} \right) d\sigma(y)$$
$$- \int_{\partial B_\epsilon(x)} \left(\Gamma \frac{\partial u}{\partial \nu} - u \frac{\partial \Gamma}{\partial \nu} \right) d\sigma(y) \ .$$

Since $\Delta \Gamma = 0$ in $D \setminus B_\epsilon(x)$, we have

$$\int_{\partial D} \left(\Gamma \frac{\partial u}{\partial \nu} - u \frac{\partial \Gamma}{\partial \nu} \right) d\sigma(y) = \int_{\partial B_\epsilon(x)} \left(\Gamma \frac{\partial u}{\partial \nu} - u \frac{\partial \Gamma}{\partial \nu} \right) d\sigma(y) \ .$$

For $d \geq 3$, we get by definition of Γ

$$\int_{\partial B_\epsilon(x)} \Gamma \frac{\partial u}{\partial \nu} \, d\sigma(y) = \frac{1}{(2-d)\omega_d} \epsilon^{2-d} \int_{\partial B_\epsilon(x)} \frac{\partial u}{\partial \nu} \, d\sigma(y) = 0$$

and

$$\int_{\partial B_\epsilon(x)} u \frac{\partial \Gamma}{\partial \nu} \, d\sigma(y) = \frac{1}{\omega_d \epsilon^{d-1}} \int_{\partial B_\epsilon(x)} u \, d\sigma(y) = u(x) \ ,$$

by the mean value property. Proceeding in the same way, we arrive at the same conclusion for $d = 2$. $\square$

3.1.2 Layer Potentials

In this subsection we show how important the fundamental solution is to potential theory. It gives rise to integral operators that invert the Laplacian. We need these integral operators (also called layer potentials) in the derivation of the decomposition theorem for solutions to the transmission problem.

Given a bounded $\mathcal{C}^2$-domain D in $\mathbb{R}^d, d \geq 2$, we denote respectively the single- and double-layer potentials of a function $\phi \in L^2(\partial D)$ as $\mathcal{S}_D \phi$ and $\mathcal{D}_D \phi$, where

$$\mathcal{S}_D \phi(x) := \int_{\partial D} \Gamma(x - y) \phi(y) \, d\sigma(y) \ , \quad x \in \mathbb{R}^d, \tag{3.5}$$

$$\mathcal{D}_D \phi(x) := \int_{\partial D} \frac{\partial}{\partial \nu_y} \Gamma(x - y) \phi(y) \, d\sigma(y) \ , \quad x \in \mathbb{R}^d \setminus \partial D \ . \tag{3.6}$$

We begin with the study of their basic properties. We note that for $x \in \mathbb{R}^d \setminus \partial D$ and $y \in \partial D$, $\partial \Gamma / \partial \nu_y (x - y)$ is an L^∞-function in y and harmonic in x, and it is $O(|x|^{1-d})$ as $|x| \to +\infty$. Therefore we readily see that $\mathcal{D}_D \phi$ and $\mathcal{S}_D \phi$ are well-defined and harmonic in $\mathbb{R}^d \setminus \partial D$. Let us list their behavior at $+\infty$.

Lemma 3.1.3 *The following holds:*

(i) $\mathcal{D}_D \phi(x) = O(|x|^{1-d})$ *as* $|x| \to +\infty$.
(ii) $\mathcal{S}_D \phi(x) = O(|x|^{2-d})$ *as* $|x| \to +\infty$ *when* $d \geq 3$.

(iii) *If $d = 2$, we have*

$$\mathcal{S}_D \phi(x) = \frac{1}{2\pi} \int_{\partial D} \phi(y)\, d\sigma(y) \ln |x| + O(|x|^{-1}) \quad \text{as } |x| \to +\infty .$$

(iv) *If $\int_{\partial D} \phi(y)\, d\sigma = 0$, then $\mathcal{S}_D \phi(x) = O(|x|^{1-d})$ as $|x| \to +\infty$ for $d \geq 2$.*

Proof. The first three properties are fairly obvious from the definitions. Let us show (iv). If $\int_{\partial D} \phi(y)\, d\sigma = 0$, then

$$\mathcal{S}_D \phi(x) = \int_{\partial D} [\Gamma(x - y) - \Gamma(x - y_0)] \phi(y) d\sigma(y) ,$$

where $y_0 \in D$. Since

$$|\Gamma(x - y) - \Gamma(x - y_0)| \leq C |x|^{1-d} \quad \text{if } |x| \to +\infty \text{ and } y \in \partial D \qquad (3.7)$$

for some constant C, $\mathcal{S}_D \phi(x) = O(|x|^{1-d})$ as $|x| \to +\infty$. $\square$

Lemma 3.1.2 now shows that if $u \in W^{1,2}(D)$ is harmonic, then for any $x \in D$,

$$u(x) = \mathcal{D}_D(u|_{\partial D}) - \mathcal{S}_D \left(\left. \frac{\partial u}{\partial \nu} \right|_{\partial D} \right) . \qquad (3.8)$$

To solve the Dirichlet and Neumann problems, where either u or $\partial u / \partial \nu$ on ∂D is unknown, we need to well-understand the subtle behaviors of the functions $\mathcal{D}_D \phi(x \pm t\nu_x)$ and $\nabla \mathcal{S}_D \phi(x \pm t\nu_x)$ for $x \in \partial D$ as $t \to 0^+$. A detailed discussion of the behavior near the boundary ∂D of $\mathcal{D}_D \phi$ and $\nabla \mathcal{S}_D \phi$ for a C^2-domain D and a density $\phi \in L^2(\partial D)$ is given below. For this purpose we shall follow [59].

Assume that D is a bounded C^2-domain. Then we have the bound

$$\left| \frac{\langle x - y, \nu_x \rangle}{|x - y|^d} \right| \leq C \frac{1}{|x - y|^{d-2}} \quad \text{for } x, y \in \partial D, x \neq y , \qquad (3.9)$$

which shows that there exists a positive constant C depending only on D such that

$$\int_{\partial D} \left(\frac{|\langle x - y, \nu_x \rangle|}{|x - y|^d} + \frac{|\langle x - y, \nu_y \rangle|}{|x - y|^d} \right) d\sigma(y) \leq C , \qquad (3.10)$$

and

$$\int_{|y - x| < \epsilon} \left(\frac{|\langle x - y, \nu_x \rangle|}{|x - y|^d} + \frac{|\langle x - y, \nu_y \rangle|}{|x - y|^d} \right) d\sigma(y) \leq C \int_0^\epsilon \frac{1}{r^{d-2}} r^{d-2}\, dr$$
$$\leq C\epsilon , \qquad (3.11)$$

for any $x \in \partial D$, by integration in polar coordinates.

Introduce the operator $\mathcal{K}_D : L^2(\partial D) \to L^2(\partial D)$ given by

$$\mathcal{K}_D\phi(x) = \frac{1}{\omega_d} \int_{\partial D} \frac{\langle y - x, \nu_y\rangle}{|x - y|^d} \phi(y)\, d\sigma(y)\,. \tag{3.12}$$

The estimate (3.10) proves that this operator is bounded. In fact, for $\phi, \psi \in L^2(\partial D)$, we estimate

$$\left| \int_{\partial D} \int_{\partial D} \frac{\langle y - x, \nu_y\rangle}{|x - y|^d} \phi(y)\, \psi(x)\, d\sigma(y)\, d\sigma(x) \right| \tag{3.13}$$

via the inequality $2ab \leq a^2 + b^2$. Then, by (3.10), (3.13) is dominated by

$$C\left(\|\phi\|^2_{L^2(\partial D)} + \|\psi\|^2_{L^2(\partial D)} \right)\,.$$

Replacing ϕ, ψ, by $t\phi, (1/t)\psi$, we see that (3.13) is bounded by

$$C\left(t^2 \|\phi\|^2_{L^2(\partial D)} + \frac{1}{t^2} \|\psi\|^2_{L^2(\partial D)} \right)\,;$$

minimizing over $t \in]0, +\infty[$, via elementary calculus, we see that (3.13) is dominated by $C\|\phi\|_{L^2(\partial D)}\|\psi\|_{L^2(\partial D)}$, proving that $\mathcal{K}_D$ is a bounded operator on $L^2(\partial D)$.

On the other hand, it is easily checked that the operator defined by

$$\mathcal{K}_D^*\phi(x) = \frac{1}{\omega_d} \int_{\partial D} \frac{\langle x - y, \nu_x\rangle}{|x - y|^d} \phi(y)\, d\sigma(y)\,, \tag{3.14}$$

is the L^2-adjoint of $\mathcal{K}_D$.

It is now important to ask about the compactness of these operators. Indeed, to apply the Fredholm theory for solving the Dirichlet and Neumann problems for the Laplace equation, we will need the following lemma.

Lemma 3.1.4 *If D is a bounded C^2-domain then the operators $\mathcal{K}_D$ and $\mathcal{K}_D^*$ are compact operators in $L^2(\partial D)$.*

Proof. It suffices to prove that $\mathcal{K}_D$ is compact in $L^2(\partial D)$ to assert that $\mathcal{K}_D^*$ is compact as well.

Given $\epsilon > 0$, set $\Gamma_\epsilon(x) = \Gamma(x)$ if $|x| > \epsilon$, $\Gamma_\epsilon(x) = 0$ otherwise, and define

$$\mathcal{K}_D^\epsilon\phi(x) = \int_{\partial D} \frac{\partial \Gamma_\epsilon}{\partial \nu_y}(x - y)\phi(y)\, d\sigma(y)\,.$$

Then

$$\int_{\partial D} \int_{\partial D} \left| \frac{\partial \Gamma_\epsilon}{\partial \nu_y}(x - y) \right|^2 d\sigma(x)\, d\sigma(y) < +\infty\,,$$

hence the operator norm of $\mathcal{K}_D^\epsilon$ on $L^2(\partial D)$ satisfies

$$\|\mathcal{K}_D^\epsilon\| \leq \left\|\frac{\partial \Gamma_\epsilon}{\partial \nu}\right\|_{L^2(\partial D \times \partial D)} .$$

Let $\{\phi_p\}_{p=1}^{+\infty}$ be an orthonormal basis for $L^2(\partial D)$. It is an easy consequence of Fubini's theorem that if $\psi_{pq}(x, y) = \phi_p(x)\phi_q(y)$, then $\{\psi_{pq}\}_{p,q=1}^{+\infty}$ is an orthonormal basis for $L^2(\partial D \times \partial D)$. Hence we can write

$$\frac{\partial \Gamma_\epsilon}{\partial \nu_y}(x - y) = \sum_{p,q=1}^{+\infty} \langle \frac{\partial \Gamma_\epsilon}{\partial \nu}, \psi_{pq} \rangle \psi_{pq}(x, y) .$$

Here $\langle, \rangle$ denotes the L^2-product. For $N \in \mathbb{N}, N \geq 2$, let

$$\mathcal{K}_D^{\epsilon,N} \phi(x) = \sum_{p+q \leq N} \int_{\partial D} \langle \frac{\partial \Gamma_\epsilon}{\partial \nu}, \psi_{pq} \rangle \psi_{pq}(x, y)\phi(y)\, d\sigma(y) .$$

It is clear that the range of $\mathcal{K}_D^{\epsilon,N}$ lies in the span of $\phi_1, \dots, \phi_N$, so $\mathcal{K}_D^{\epsilon,N}$ is of finite rank. Moreover

$$\left\|\mathcal{K}_D^\epsilon - \mathcal{K}_D^{\epsilon,N}\right\| \leq \left\|\frac{\partial \Gamma_\epsilon}{\partial \nu} - \sum_{p+q \leq N} \langle \frac{\partial \Gamma_\epsilon}{\partial \nu}, \psi_{pq} \rangle \psi_{pq}\right\|_{L^2(\partial D \times \partial D)} \longrightarrow 0 \quad \text{as } N \to +\infty,$$

and then $\mathcal{K}_D^\epsilon$ is compact. On the other hand,

$$\mathcal{K}_D\phi(x) = \frac{1}{\omega_d}\int_{|y-x|>\epsilon} \frac{\langle y - x, \nu_y \rangle}{|x - y|^d}\phi(y)\, d\sigma(y)$$

$$+ \frac{1}{\omega_d}\int_{|y-x|<\epsilon} \frac{\langle y - x, \nu_y \rangle}{|x - y|^d}\phi(y)\, d\sigma(y) ,$$

$$= \mathcal{K}_D^\epsilon\phi(x) + \frac{1}{\omega_d}\int_{|y-x|<\epsilon} \frac{\langle y - x, \nu_y \rangle}{|x - y|^d}\phi(y)\, d\sigma(y) ,$$

and then, by the estimate (3.11) the operator norm of $\mathcal{K}_D - \mathcal{K}_D^\epsilon$ tends to zero as $\epsilon \to 0$, so $\mathcal{K}_D$ is compact. $\square$

In the special case of the unit sphere, we may simplify the expressions defining the operators $\mathcal{K}_D$ and $\mathcal{K}_D^*$.

Lemma 3.1.5 (i) *Suppose that D is a two dimensional disk with radius r. Then,*

$$\frac{\langle x - y, \nu_x \rangle}{|x - y|^2} = \frac{1}{2r} \quad \forall\, x, y \in \partial D, x \neq y ,$$

and therefore, for any $\phi \in L^2(\partial D)$,

$$\mathcal{K}_D^*\phi(x) = \mathcal{K}_D\phi(x) = \frac{1}{4\pi r}\int_{\partial D} \phi(y)\, d\sigma(y) , \tag{3.15}$$

for all $x \in \partial D$.

(ii) *For $d \geq 3$, if D denotes a sphere with radius r, then, since*

$$\frac{\langle x - y, \nu_x \rangle}{|x - y|^d} = \frac{1}{2r} \frac{1}{|x - y|^{d-2}} \quad \forall\, x, y \in \partial D, x \neq y,$$

we have that for any $\phi \in L^2(\partial D)$,

$$\mathcal{K}_D^* \phi(x) = \mathcal{K}_D \phi(x) = \frac{(2 - d)}{2r} \mathcal{S}_D \phi(x) \tag{3.16}$$

for any $x \in \partial D$.

Turning now to the behavior of the double layer potential at the boundary, we first establish that the double layer potential with constant density has a jump.

Lemma 3.1.6 *If D is a bounded $\mathcal{C}^2$-domain then $\mathcal{D}_D(1)(x) = 0$ for $x \in \mathbb{R}^d \setminus \overline{D}$, $\mathcal{D}_D(1)(x) = 1$ for $x \in D$, and $\mathcal{K}_D(1)(x) = 1/2$ for $x \in \partial D$.*

Proof. The first equation follows immediately from Green's formula, since $\Gamma(x - y)$ is in $\mathcal{C}^\infty(\overline{D})$ and harmonic in D as a function of y when $x \in \mathbb{R}^d \setminus \overline{D}$. As for the second equation, given $x \in D$, let $\epsilon > 0$ be small enough so that $\overline{B_\epsilon} \subset D$, where B_ϵ is the ball of center x and radius ϵ. We can apply Green's formula to $\Gamma(x - y)$ on the domain $D \setminus \overline{B_\epsilon}$ to obtain

$$0 = \mathcal{D}_D(1)(x) - \frac{\epsilon^{1-d}}{\omega_d} \int_{\partial B_\epsilon} d\sigma(y)$$
$$= \mathcal{D}_D(1)(x) - 1.$$

Now we prove the third equation. Given $x \in \partial D$, again let B_ϵ be the ball of center x and radius ϵ. Set $\partial D_\epsilon = \partial D \setminus (\partial D \cap B_\epsilon)$, $\partial B'_\epsilon = \partial B_\epsilon \cap D$, and $\partial B''_\epsilon = \{y \in \partial B_\epsilon : \nu_x \cdot y < 0\}$. (Thus $\partial B''_\epsilon$ is the hemisphere of ∂B_ϵ lying on the same side of the tangent plane to ∂D at x.) A further application of Green's formula shows that

$$0 = \frac{1}{\omega_d} \int_{\partial D_\epsilon} \frac{\langle y - x, \nu_y \rangle}{|x - y|^d} d\sigma(y) + \int_{\partial B'_\epsilon} \frac{\partial \Gamma}{\partial \nu_y} (x - y)\, d\sigma(y).$$

Thus

$$\frac{1}{\omega_d} \int_{\partial D_\epsilon} \frac{\langle y - x, \nu_y \rangle}{|x - y|^d} d\sigma(y) = -\int_{\partial B'_\epsilon} \frac{\partial \Gamma}{\partial \nu_y} (x - y)\, d\sigma(y) = \frac{\epsilon^{1-d}}{\omega_d} \int_{\partial B'_\epsilon} d\sigma(y).$$

But on the one hand, clearly

$$\int_{\partial D} \frac{\langle y - x, \nu_y \rangle}{|x - y|^d} d\sigma(y) = \lim_{\epsilon \to 0} \int_{\partial D_\epsilon} \frac{\langle y - x, \nu_y \rangle}{|x - y|^d} d\sigma(y).$$

On the other hand, since ∂D is $\mathcal{C}^2$, the distance between the tangent plane to ∂D at x and the points on ∂D at a distance ϵ from x is $O(\epsilon^2)$, so

$$\int_{\partial B'_\epsilon} d\sigma(y) = \int_{\partial B''_\epsilon} d\sigma(y) + O(\epsilon^2) \cdot O(\epsilon^{d-1}) = \frac{\omega_d \epsilon^{d-1}}{2} + O(\epsilon^{d+1}) ,$$

and the desired result follows. $\square$

Lemma 3.1.6 can be extended to general densities $\phi \in L^2(\partial D)$. For convenience we introduce the following notation. For a function u defined on $\mathbb{R}^d \setminus \partial D$, we denote

$$u|_\pm(x) := \lim_{t \to 0^+} u(x \pm t\nu_x), \quad x \in \partial D ,$$

and

$$\left. \frac{\partial}{\partial \nu_x} u \right|_\pm (x) := \lim_{t \to 0^+} \langle \nabla u(x \pm t\nu_x), \nu_x \rangle , \quad x \in \partial D ,$$

if the limits exist. Here ν_x is the outward unit normal to ∂D at x, and $\langle , \rangle$ denotes the scalar product in $\mathbb{R}^d$. For ease of notation we will sometimes use the dot for the scalar product in $\mathbb{R}^d$.

We relate in the next lemma the traces $\mathcal{D}_D|_\pm$ of the double-layer potential to the operator $\mathcal{K}_D$ defined by (3.12).

Lemma 3.1.7 *If D is a bounded $\mathcal{C}^2$-domain then for $\phi \in L^2(\partial D)$*

$$(\mathcal{D}_D \phi)|_\pm (x) = \left(\mp \frac{1}{2} I + \mathcal{K}_D \right) \phi(x) \quad a.e. \ x \in \partial D . \tag{3.17}$$

Proof. First we consider a density $f \in \mathcal{C}^0(\partial D)$. If $x \in \partial D$ and $t < 0$ is sufficiently small, then $x + t\nu_x \in D$, so by Lemma 3.1.6,

$$\mathcal{D}_D f(x + t\nu_x) = f(x) + \int_{\partial D} \frac{\partial \Gamma}{\partial \nu_y}(x + t\nu_x - y)(f(y) - f(x)) \, d\sigma(y) . \tag{3.18}$$

To prove that the second integral is continuous as $t \to 0^-$, given $\epsilon > 0$ let $\delta > 0$ be such that $|f(y) - f(x)| < \epsilon$ whenever $|y - x| < \delta$.

Then

$$\int_{\partial D} \frac{\partial \Gamma}{\partial \nu_y}(x + t\nu_x - y)(f(y) - f(x)) \, d\sigma(y) - \int_{\partial D} \frac{\partial \Gamma}{\partial \nu_y}(x - y)(f(y) - f(x)) \, d\sigma(y)$$

$$= \int_{\partial D \cap B_\delta} \frac{\partial \Gamma}{\partial \nu_y}(x + t\nu_x - y)(f(y) - f(x)) \, d\sigma(y)$$

$$- \int_{\partial D \cap B_\delta} \frac{\partial \Gamma}{\partial \nu_y}(x - y)(f(y) - f(x)) \, d\sigma(y)$$

$$+ \int_{\partial D \setminus B_\delta} \left(\frac{\partial \Gamma}{\partial \nu_y}(x + t\nu_x - y) - \frac{\partial \Gamma}{\partial \nu_y}(x - y) \right)(f(y) - f(x)) \, d\sigma(y)$$

$$= I_1 + I_2 + I_3 .$$

Here B_δ is the ball of center x and radius δ. It easily follows from (3.10) that $|I_2| \leq C\epsilon$. Since

$$\left| \frac{\partial \Gamma}{\partial \nu_y}(x + t\nu_x - y) - \frac{\partial \Gamma}{\partial \nu_y}(x - y) \right| \leq C\frac{|t|}{|x-y|^d} \quad \forall\, y \in \partial D,$$

we get $|I_3| \leq CM|t|$, where M is the maximum of f on ∂D. To estimate I_1, we assume that $x = 0$ and near the origin, D is given by $y = (y', y_d)$ with $y_d > \varphi(y')$, where φ is a C^2-function such that $\varphi(0) = 0$ and $\nabla\varphi(0) = 0$. With the local coordinates, we can show that

$$\left| \frac{\partial \Gamma}{\partial \nu_y}(x + t\nu_x - y) \right| \leq C\frac{|\varphi(y')| + |t|}{(|y'|^2 + |t|^2)^{d/2}},$$

and hence $|I_1| \leq C\epsilon$. A combination of the above estimates yields

$$\limsup_{t \to 0^-} \left| \int_{\partial D} \frac{\partial \Gamma}{\partial \nu_y}(x + t\nu_x - y)(f(y) - f(x))\, d\sigma(y) \right.$$
$$\left. - \int_{\partial D} \frac{\partial \Gamma}{\partial \nu_y}(x - y)(f(y) - f(x)\, d\sigma(y) \right| \leq C\epsilon.$$

Since ϵ is arbitrary, we obtain that

$$(\mathcal{D}_D f)\big|_-(x) = f(x) + \int_{\partial D} \frac{\partial \Gamma}{\partial \nu_y}(x - y)(f(y) - f(x))\, d\sigma(y)$$
$$= \left(\frac{1}{2}I + \mathcal{K}_D \right) f(x) \quad \text{for } x \in \partial D.$$

If $t > 0$, the argument is the same except that

$$\int_{\partial D} \frac{\partial \Gamma}{\partial \nu_y}(x + t\nu_x - y)\, d\sigma(y) = 0,$$

and hence we write

$$\mathcal{D}_D f(x + t\nu_x) = \int_{\partial D} \frac{\partial \Gamma}{\partial \nu_y}(x + t\nu_x - y)(f(y) - f(x))\, d\sigma(y), \quad x \in \partial D,$$

instead of (3.18). We leave the rest of the proof to the reader.

Next, consider $\phi \in L^2(\partial D)$. We first note that by (3.10), $\lim_{t\to 0^+} \mathcal{D}_D \phi(x \pm t\nu_x)$ exists and

$$\left\| \limsup_{t \to 0^+} \mathcal{D}_D \phi(x \pm t\nu_x) \right\|_{L^2(\partial D)} \leq C\|\phi\|_{L^2(\partial D)},$$

for some positive constant C independent of ϕ.

To handle the general case, let ϵ be given and choose a function $f \in C^0(\partial D)$ satisfying $\|\phi - f\|_{L^2(\partial D)} < \epsilon$.

Then

$$\left| \mathcal{D}_D\phi(x \pm t\nu_x) - \left(\mp \frac{1}{2}I + \mathcal{K}_D \right)\phi(x) \right|$$

$$\leq \left| \mathcal{D}_D f(x \pm t\nu_x) - \left(\mp \frac{1}{2}I + \mathcal{K}_D \right)f(x) \right| + \left| \mathcal{D}_D(\phi - f)(x \pm t\nu_x) \right|$$

$$+ \left| \left(\mp \frac{1}{2}I + \mathcal{K}_D \right)(\phi - f)(x) \right| .$$

For $\lambda > 0$, let

$$A_\lambda = \left\{ x \in \partial D : \limsup_{t \to 0^+} \left| \mathcal{D}_D\phi(x \pm t\nu_x) - (\mp \frac{1}{2}I + \mathcal{K}_D)\phi(x) \right| > \lambda \right\} .$$

For a set E let $|E|$ denote its Lebesgue measure. Then

$$|A_\lambda| \leq \left| \left\{ |\mathcal{D}_D(\phi - f)| > \frac{\lambda}{3} \right\} \right| + \left| \left\{ |\phi - f| > \frac{2\lambda}{3} \right\} \right| + \left| \left\{ |\mathcal{K}_D(\phi - f)| > \frac{\lambda}{3} \right\} \right|$$

$$\leq (\frac{3}{\lambda})^2 \left(\|\phi - f\|^2_{L^2(\partial D)} + \frac{1}{4}\|\phi - f\|^2_{L^2(\partial D)} + \|\mathcal{K}_D(\phi - f)\|^2_{L^2(\partial D)} \right)$$

$$\leq C(\frac{3}{\lambda})^2 \epsilon^2 .$$

Here we have used the L^2-boundedness of $\mathcal{K}_D$ which is an obvious consequence of Lemma 3.1.4. Since ϵ is arbitrary, $|A_\lambda| = 0$ for all $\lambda > 0$. This implies that

$$\lim_{t \to 0^+} \mathcal{D}_D\phi(x \pm t\nu_x) = (\mp \frac{1}{2}I + \mathcal{K}_D)\phi(x) \quad \text{a.e. } x \in \partial D ,$$

and completes the proof. □

In a similar way, we can describe the behavior of the gradient of the single layer potential at the boundary. The following lemma reveals the connection between the traces $\partial \mathcal{S}_D/\partial\nu|_\pm$ and the operator $\mathcal{K}_D^*$ defined by (3.14).

Lemma 3.1.8 *If D is a bounded C^2-domain then for $\phi \in L^2(\partial D)$:*

$$\frac{\partial}{\partial T}\mathcal{S}_D\phi \bigg|_+ (x) = \frac{\partial}{\partial T}\mathcal{S}_D\phi \bigg|_- (x) \quad \text{a.e. } x \in \partial D , \tag{3.19}$$

and

$$\frac{\partial}{\partial\nu}\mathcal{S}_D\phi \bigg|_\pm (x) = \left(\pm\frac{1}{2}I + \mathcal{K}_D^* \right)\phi(x) \quad \text{a.e. } x \in \partial D . \tag{3.20}$$

Consider now the integral equations

$$\left(\frac{I}{2} + \mathcal{K}_D \right)\phi = f \quad \text{and} \quad \left(\frac{I}{2} - \mathcal{K}_D^* \right)\psi = g , \tag{3.21}$$

for $f, g \in L^2(\partial D), \int_{\partial D} g \, d\sigma = 0$.

By the trace formulae (3.20) and (3.17) for the single- and double-layer potentials, it is easily seen that if ϕ and ψ are solutions to these equations then $\mathcal{D}_D\phi$ solves the Dirichlet problem with Dirichlet data f and $-\mathcal{S}_D\psi$ solves the Neumann problem with Neumann data g.

In view of Lemma 3.1.4, we can apply the Fredholm theory to study the solvability of the two integral equations in (3.21).

3.1.3 Invertibility of $\lambda I - \mathcal{K}_D^*$

Let now D be a bounded domain, and let

$$L_0^2(\partial D) := \left\{ \phi \in L^2(\partial D) : \int_{\partial D} \phi \, d\sigma = 0 \right\} .$$

Let $\lambda \neq 0$ be a real number. Of particular interest for solving the transmission problem for the Laplacian would be the invertibility of the operator $\lambda I - \mathcal{K}_D^*$ on $L^2(\partial D)$ or $L_0^2(\partial D)$ for $|\lambda| \geq 1/2$. The case $|\lambda| = 1/2$ corresponds to the integral equations in (3.21).

To further motivate this subsection, suppose that D has conductivity $0 < k \neq 1 < +\infty$. Consider the transmission problem

$$\begin{cases} \nabla \cdot \left(1 + (k-1)\chi(D)\right)\nabla u = 0 & \text{in } \mathbb{R}^d , \\ u(x) - H(x) \to 0 & \text{as } |x| \to +\infty , \end{cases}$$

where H is a harmonic function. It can be shown that this problem can be reduced to solving the integral equation

$$(\lambda I - \mathcal{K}_D^*)\phi = \frac{\partial H}{\partial \nu} \quad \text{on } \partial D .$$

First, it was proved by Kellog in [79] that the eigenvalues of $\mathcal{K}_D^*$ on $L^2(\partial D)$ lie in $]-1/2, 1/2]$. The following injectivity result holds.

Lemma 3.1.9 *Let λ be a real number and let D be a bounded C^2-domain. The operator $\lambda I - \mathcal{K}_D^*$ is one to one on $L_0^2(\partial D)$ if $|\lambda| \geq 1/2$, and for $\lambda \in]-\infty, -1/2] \cup]1/2, +\infty[$, $\lambda I - \mathcal{K}_D^*$ is one to one on $L^2(\partial D)$.*

Proof. The argument is by contradiction. Let $\lambda \in]-\infty, -1/2] \cup]1/2, +\infty[$, and assume that $\phi \in L^2(\partial D)$ satisfies $(\lambda I - \mathcal{K}_D^*)\phi = 0$ and ϕ is not identically zero. Since $\mathcal{K}_D(1) = 1/2$ by Green's formula, we have

$$0 = \int_{\partial D} (\lambda I - \mathcal{K}_D^*)\phi \, d\sigma = \int_{\partial D} \phi(\lambda - \mathcal{K}_D(1)) \, d\sigma$$

and thus $\int_{\partial D} \phi \, d\sigma = 0$. Hence $\mathcal{S}_D\phi(x) = O(|x|^{1-d})$ and $\nabla\mathcal{S}_D\phi(x) = O(|x|^{-d})$ at infinity for $d \geq 2$. Since ϕ is not identically zero, both of the following numbers cannot be zero:

$$A = \int_D |\nabla \mathcal{S}_D \phi|^2 \, dx \text{ and } B = \int_{\mathbb{R}^d \setminus \overline{D}} |\nabla \mathcal{S}_D \phi|^2 \, dx \ .$$

In fact, if both of them are zero, then $\mathcal{S}_D \phi = $ constant in D and in $\mathbb{R}^d \setminus \overline{D}$. Hence $\phi = 0$ by

$$\left. \frac{\partial}{\partial \nu} \mathcal{S}_D \phi \right|_+ - \left. \frac{\partial}{\partial \nu} \mathcal{S}_D \phi \right|_- = \phi \quad \text{on } \partial D,$$

which is a contradiction.

On the other hand, using the divergence theorem and (3.20), we have

$$A = \int_{\partial D} (-\frac{1}{2} I + \mathcal{K}_D^*) \phi \, \mathcal{S}_D \phi \, d\sigma \text{ and } B = -\int_{\partial D} (\frac{1}{2} I + \mathcal{K}_D^*) \phi \, \mathcal{S}_D \phi \, d\sigma \ .$$

Since $(\lambda I - \mathcal{K}_D^*) \phi = 0$, it follows that

$$\lambda = \frac{1}{2} \frac{B - A}{B + A} \ .$$

Thus, $|\lambda| < 1/2$, which is a contradiction and so, for $\lambda \in]-\infty, -\frac{1}{2}] \cup [\frac{1}{2}, +\infty[$, $\lambda I - \mathcal{K}_D^*$ is one to one on $L^2(\partial D)$.

If $\lambda = 1/2$, then $A = 0$ and hence $\mathcal{S}_D \phi = $ constant in D. Thus $\mathcal{S}_D \phi$ is harmonic in $\mathbb{R}^d \setminus \partial D$, behaves like $O(|x|^{1-d})$ as $|x| \to +\infty$ (since $\phi \in L_0^2(\partial D)$), and is constant on ∂D. By (3.20), we have $\mathcal{K}_D^* \phi = (1/2) \phi$, and hence

$$B = -\int_{\partial D} \phi \, \mathcal{S}_D \phi \, d\sigma = C \int_{\partial D} \phi \, d\sigma = 0 \ ,$$

which forces us to conclude that $\phi = 0$. This proves that $(1/2) I - \mathcal{K}_D^*$ is one to one on $L_0^2(\partial D)$. $\square$

Let us now turn to the surjectivity of the operator $\lambda I - \mathcal{K}_D^*$ on $L^2(\partial D)$ or $L_0^2(\partial D)$. Since D is a bounded $\mathcal{C}^2$-domain then, as shown in Lemma 3.1.4, the operators $\mathcal{K}_D$ and $\mathcal{K}_D^*$ are compact operators in $L^2(\partial D)$. Therefore, the surjectivity of $\lambda I - \mathcal{K}_D^*$ holds, by applying the Fredholm alternative.

3.1.4 Neumann Function

Let Ω be a smooth bounded domain in $\mathbb{R}^d, d \geq 2$. Let $N(x, z)$ be the Neumann function for $-\Delta$ in Ω corresponding to a Dirac mass at z. That is, N is the solution to

$$\begin{cases} -\Delta_x N(x, z) = \delta_z & \text{in } \Omega \ , \\ \left. \frac{\partial N}{\partial \nu_x} \right|_{\partial \Omega} = -\frac{1}{|\partial \Omega|} \ , \int_{\partial \Omega} N(x, z) \, d\sigma(x) = 0 & \text{for } z \in \Omega \ . \end{cases} \tag{3.22}$$

Note that the Neumann function $N(x, z)$ is defined as a function of $x \in \overline{\Omega}$ for each fixed $z \in \Omega$.

The operator defined by $N(x, z)$ is the solution operator for the Neumann problem

$$\begin{cases} \Delta U = 0 & \text{in } \Omega , \\ \dfrac{\partial U}{\partial \nu}\Big|_{\partial \Omega} = g , \end{cases} \tag{3.23}$$

namely, the function U defined by

$$U(x) := \int_{\partial \Omega} N(x, z)g(z)\,d\sigma(z)$$

is the solution to (3.23) satisfying $\int_{\partial \Omega} U\,d\sigma = 0$.

Now we discuss some properties of N as a function of x and z.

Lemma 3.1.10 (Neumann Function) *The Neumann function N is symmetric in its arguments, that is, $N(x, z) = N(z, x)$ for $x \neq z \in \Omega$. Furthermore, it has the form*

$$N(x, z) = \begin{cases} -\dfrac{1}{2\pi} \ln |x - z| + R_2(x, z) & \text{if } d = 2 , \\ \dfrac{1}{(d-2)\omega_d} \dfrac{1}{|x-z|^{d-2}} + R_d(x, z) & \text{if } d \geq 3 , \end{cases} \tag{3.24}$$

where $R_d(\cdot, z)$ belongs to $W^{\frac{3}{2}, 2}(\Omega)$ for any $z \in \Omega, d \geq 2$ and solves

$$\begin{cases} \Delta_x R_d(x, z) = 0 & \text{in } \Omega , \\ \dfrac{\partial R_d}{\partial \nu_x}\Big|_{\partial \Omega} = -\dfrac{1}{|\partial \Omega|} + \dfrac{1}{\omega_d} \dfrac{\langle x - z, \nu_x \rangle}{|x - z|^d} & \text{for } x \in \partial \Omega . \end{cases}$$

Proof. Pick $z_1, z_2 \in \Omega$ with $z_1 \neq z_2$. Let $B_r(z_p) = \{|x - z_p| < r\}$, $p = 1, 2$. Choose $r > 0$ so small that $B_r(z_1) \cap B_r(z_2) = \emptyset$. Set $N_1(x) = N(x, z_1)$ and $N_2(x) = N(x, z_2)$. We apply Green's formula in $\Omega' = \Omega \setminus B_r(z_1) \cup B_r(z_2)$ to get

$$\int_{\Omega'} \left(N_1 \Delta N_2 - N_2 \Delta N_1 \right) dx = \int_{\partial \Omega} \left(N_1 \frac{\partial N_2}{\partial \nu} - N_2 \frac{\partial N_1}{\partial \nu} \right) d\sigma$$
$$- \int_{\partial B_r(z_1)} \left(N_1 \frac{\partial N_2}{\partial \nu} - N_2 \frac{\partial N_1}{\partial \nu} \right) d\sigma - \int_{\partial B_r(z_2)} \left(N_1 \frac{\partial N_2}{\partial \nu} - N_2 \frac{\partial N_1}{\partial \nu} \right) d\sigma ,$$

where all the derivatives are with respect to the x–variable with z fixed. Since N_p, $p = 1, 2$, is harmonic for $x \neq z_p$, $\partial N_1/\partial \nu = \partial N_2/\partial \nu = -1/|\partial \Omega|$, and $\int_{\partial \Omega}(N_1 - N_2)\,d\sigma = 0$, we have

$$\int_{\partial B_r(z_1)} \left(N_1 \frac{\partial N_2}{\partial \nu} - N_2 \frac{\partial N_1}{\partial \nu} \right) d\sigma + \int_{\partial B_r(z_2)} \left(N_1 \frac{\partial N_2}{\partial \nu} - N_2 \frac{\partial N_1}{\partial \nu} \right) d\sigma = 0 .$$
$$\tag{3.25}$$

Thanks to (3.24) which will be proved shortly, the left-hand side of (3.25) has the same limit as $r \to 0$ as the left-hand side of the following identity:

$$\int_{\partial B_r(z_1)} \left(\Gamma \frac{\partial N_2}{\partial \nu} - N_2 \frac{\partial \Gamma}{\partial \nu} \right) d\sigma + \int_{\partial B_r(z_2)} \left(N_1 \frac{\partial \Gamma}{\partial \nu} - \Gamma \frac{\partial N_1}{\partial \nu} \right) d\sigma = 0 .$$

Since

$$\int_{\partial B_r(z_1)} \Gamma \frac{\partial N_2}{\partial \nu} d\sigma \to 0 , \quad \int_{\partial B_r(z_2)} \Gamma \frac{\partial N_1}{\partial \nu} d\sigma \to 0 \quad \text{as } r \to 0 ,$$

and

$$\int_{\partial B_r(z_1)} N_2 \frac{\partial \Gamma}{\partial \nu} d\sigma \to N_2(z_1) , \quad \int_{\partial B_r(z_2)} N_1 \frac{\partial \Gamma}{\partial \nu} d\sigma \to N_1(z_2) \quad \text{as } r \to 0 ,$$

we obtain $N_2(z_1) - N_1(z_2) = 0$, or equivalently $N(z_2, z_1) = N(z_1, z_2)$ for any $z_1 \neq z_2 \in \Omega$.

Now let $R_d, d \geq 2$, be defined by

$$R_d(x, z) = \begin{cases} N(x, z) + \dfrac{1}{2\pi} \ln |x - z| & \text{if } d = 2 , \\ N(x, z) + \dfrac{1}{(2 - d)\omega_d} \dfrac{1}{|x - z|^{d-2}} & \text{if } d \geq 3 . \end{cases}$$

Since $R_d(\cdot, z)$ is harmonic in Ω and $\partial R_d(\cdot, z)/\partial \nu \in L^2(\partial \Omega)$, it follows from the standard elliptic regularity theory that $R_d(\cdot, z) \in W^{\frac{3}{2}, 2}(\Omega)$ for any $z \in \Omega$. □

Note that, because of (3.24), the formula

$$U(x) \approx -\mathcal{S}_\Omega g \quad \text{in } \Omega ,$$

has been proposed as a first approximation of the solution to the Neumann problem (3.23).

For D, a subset of Ω, let

$$N_D f(x) := \int_{\partial D} N(x, y) f(y) \, d\sigma(y), \quad x \in \Omega .$$

The following lemma relates the fundamental solution Γ to the Neumann function N.

Lemma 3.1.11 *For $z \in \Omega$ and $x \in \partial \Omega$, let $\Gamma_z(x) := \Gamma(x - z)$ and $N_z(x) := N(x, z)$. Then*

$$\left(-\frac{1}{2} I + \mathcal{K}_\Omega \right)(N_z)(x) = \Gamma_z(x) \quad \text{modulo constants}, \quad x \in \partial \Omega , \qquad (3.26)$$

or, to be more precise, for any simply connected smooth domain D compactly contained in Ω and for any $g \in L_0^2(\partial D)$, we have for any $x \in \partial \Omega$

$$\int_{\partial D} \left(-\frac{1}{2}I + \mathcal{K}_\Omega \right) (N_z)(x) g(z)\, d\sigma(z) = \int_{\partial D} \Gamma_z(x) g(z)\, d\sigma(z)\,, \qquad (3.27)$$

or equivalently,

$$\left(-\frac{1}{2}I + \mathcal{K}_\Omega \right) \left((N_D g)\big|_{\partial\Omega} \right)(x) = \mathcal{S}_D g(x)\,. \qquad (3.28)$$

Proof.   Let $f \in L_0^2(\partial\Omega)$ and define

$$u(z) := \int_{\partial\Omega} \left(-\frac{1}{2}I + \mathcal{K}_\Omega \right)(N_z)(x) f(x)\, d\sigma(x), \quad z \in \Omega\,.$$

Then

$$u(z) = \int_{\partial\Omega} N(x, z) \left(-\frac{1}{2}I + \mathcal{K}_\Omega^* \right) f(x)\, d\sigma(x)\,.$$

Therefore, $\Delta u = 0$ in Ω and

$$\left. \frac{\partial u}{\partial \nu} \right|_{\partial\Omega} = (-\frac{1}{2}I + \mathcal{K}_\Omega^*) f\,.$$

Hence by the uniqueness modulo constants of a solution to the Neumann problem we have

$$u(z) - \mathcal{S}_\Omega f(z) = \text{constant}, \quad z \in \Omega\,.$$

Thus if $g \in L_0^2(\partial D)$, we obtain

$$\int_{\partial\Omega} \int_{\partial D} \left(-\frac{1}{2}I + \mathcal{K}_\Omega \right)(N_z)(x) g(z) f(x)\, d\sigma(z)\, d\sigma(x)$$

$$= \int_{\partial\Omega} \int_{\partial D} \Gamma_z(x) g(z) f(x)\, d\sigma(z)\, d\sigma(x)\,.$$

Since f is arbitrary, we have equation (3.26) or, equivalently, (3.27). This completes the proof.   □

The following simple observation is useful.

Lemma 3.1.12 Let $f \in L^2(\partial\Omega)$ satisfy $\left(\frac{1}{2}I - \mathcal{K}_\Omega \right) f = 0$. Then f is constant.

Proof.   Let $f \in L^2(\partial\Omega)$ be such that $((1/2)I - \mathcal{K}_\Omega) f = 0$. Then for any $g \in L^2(\partial\Omega)$

$$\int_{\partial\Omega} (\frac{1}{2}I - \mathcal{K}_\Omega) f(x) g(x)\, d\sigma(x) = 0\,,$$

or equivalently,

$$\int_{\partial\Omega} f(x)(\frac{1}{2}I - \mathcal{K}_\Omega^*) g(x)\, d\sigma(x) = 0\,.$$

But $\text{Range}((1/2)I - \mathcal{K}_\Omega^*) = L_0^2(\partial\Omega)$ and so, f is constant.   □

We mention that the Neumann function for the ball $B_R(0)$ is given, for any $x, z \in B_R(0)$, by

$$N(x, z) = \frac{1}{4\pi|x - z|} + \frac{1}{4\pi\left|\frac{R}{|x|}x - \frac{|x|}{R}z\right|}$$

$$+ \frac{1}{4\pi R}\ln\frac{2}{1 - \frac{x \cdot z}{R^2} + \frac{1}{R}\left|\frac{|x|}{R}z - \frac{R}{|x|}x\right|} - \frac{1}{2\pi R} \quad \text{for } d = 3 , \tag{3.29}$$

and by

$$N(x, z) = -\frac{1}{2\pi}\left(\ln|x - z| + \ln\left|\frac{R}{|x|}x - \frac{|x|}{R}z\right|\right) + \frac{\ln R}{\pi} \quad \text{for } d = 2 . \tag{3.30}$$

3.1.5 Transmission Problem

Let Ω be a bounded domain in $\mathbb{R}^d$ with a connected smooth boundary and conductivity equal to 1. Consider a bounded domain $D \subset\subset \Omega$ with a connected smooth boundary and conductivity $0 < k \neq 1 < +\infty$.

Let $g \in L_0^2(\partial\Omega)$, and let u and U be respectively the (variational) solutions of the Neumann problems

$$\begin{cases} \nabla \cdot \left(1 + (k - 1)\chi(D)\right)\nabla u = 0 & \text{in } \Omega , \\ \left.\dfrac{\partial u}{\partial \nu}\right|_{\partial\Omega} = g , \\ \displaystyle\int_{\partial\Omega} u(x)\, d\sigma(x) = 0 , \end{cases} \tag{3.31}$$

and

$$\begin{cases} \Delta U = 0 & \text{in } \Omega , \\ \left.\dfrac{\partial U}{\partial \nu}\right|_{\partial\Omega} = g , \\ \displaystyle\int_{\partial\Omega} U(x)\, d\sigma(x) = 0 , \end{cases} \tag{3.32}$$

where $\chi(D)$ is the characteristic function of D. Clearly, the Lax-Milgram lemma shows that, given $g \in L_0^2(\partial\Omega)$, there exist unique u and U in $W^{1,2}(\Omega)$ which solve (3.31) and (3.32).

At this point we have all the necessary ingredients to state a decomposition formula of the steady-state voltage potential u into a harmonic part and a refraction part. This decomposition formula is unique and seems to inherit geometric properties of the anomaly D. We refer to [13] for its proof.

Theorem 3.1.13 (Decomposition Formula) *Suppose that D is a domain compactly contained in Ω with a connected smooth boundary and conductivity $0 < k \neq 1 < +\infty$. Then the solution u of the Neumann problem (3.31) is represented as*

$$u(x) = H(x) + \mathcal{S}_D\phi(x), \quad x \in \Omega, \tag{3.33}$$

where the harmonic function H is given by

$$H(x) = -\mathcal{S}_\Omega(g)(x) + \mathcal{D}_\Omega(f)(x), \quad x \in \Omega, \quad f := u|_{\partial\Omega} \in W^2_{\frac{1}{2}}(\partial\Omega), \tag{3.34}$$

and $\phi \in L^2_0(\partial D)$ satisfies the integral equation

$$\left(\frac{k+1}{2(k-1)}I - \mathcal{K}^*_D\right)\phi = \frac{\partial H}{\partial\nu}\bigg|_{\partial D} \quad on \ \partial D. \tag{3.35}$$

The decomposition (3.33) into a harmonic part and a refraction part is unique. Moreover, $\forall\, n \in \mathbb{N}$, there exists a constant $C_n = C(n, \Omega, \mathrm{dist}(D, \partial\Omega))$ independent of D and the conductivity k such that

$$\|H\|_{\mathcal{C}^n(\overline{D})} \leq C_n\|g\|_{L^2(\partial\Omega)}. \tag{3.36}$$

Furthermore, the following holds

$$H(x) + \mathcal{S}_D\phi(x) = 0, \quad \forall\, x \in \mathbb{R}^d \setminus \overline{\Omega}. \tag{3.37}$$

Another useful expression of the harmonic part H of u is given in the following lemma.

Lemma 3.1.14 *We have*

$$H(x) = \begin{cases} u(x) - (k-1)\displaystyle\int_D \nabla_y\Gamma(x-y)\cdot\nabla u(y)\,dy, & x \in \Omega, \\[4mm] -(k-1)\displaystyle\int_D \nabla_y\Gamma(x-y)\cdot\nabla u(y)\,dy, & x \in \mathbb{R}^d\setminus\overline{\Omega}. \end{cases} \tag{3.38}$$

Proof. We claim that

$$\phi = (k-1)\frac{\partial u}{\partial\nu}\bigg|_-. \tag{3.39}$$

In fact, it follows from the jump formula (3.20) and the equations (3.33) and (3.35) that

$$\frac{\partial u}{\partial\nu}\bigg|_- = \frac{\partial H}{\partial\nu} + \frac{\partial}{\partial\nu}\mathcal{S}_D\phi\bigg|_- = \frac{\partial H}{\partial\nu} + (-\frac{1}{2}I + \mathcal{K}^*_D)\phi = \frac{1}{k-1}\phi \quad on \ \partial D.$$

Then (3.38) follows from (3.37) and (3.39) by Green's formula. $\quad\square$

Let $g \in L_0^2(\partial\Omega)$ and

$$U(y) := \int_{\partial\Omega} N(x, y) g(x) \, d\sigma(x) .$$

Then U is the solution to the Neumann problem (3.32) and the following representation holds.

Theorem 3.1.15 *The solution u of (3.31) can be represented as*

$$u(x) = U(x) - N_D \phi(x), \quad x \in \partial\Omega , \tag{3.40}$$

where ϕ is defined in (3.35).

Proof. By substituting (3.33) into (3.34), we obtain

$$H(x) = -\mathcal{S}_\Omega(g)(x) + \mathcal{D}_\Omega \Big(H|_{\partial\Omega} + (\mathcal{S}_D \phi)|_{\partial\Omega} \Big)(x), \quad x \in \Omega .$$

It then follows from (3.17) that

$$\Big(\frac{1}{2}I - \mathcal{K}_\Omega\Big)(H|_{\partial\Omega}) = -(\mathcal{S}_\Omega g)|_{\partial\Omega} + \Big(\frac{1}{2}I + \mathcal{K}_\Omega\Big)((\mathcal{S}_D \phi)|_{\partial\Omega}) \quad \text{on } \partial\Omega . \tag{3.41}$$

Since $U = -\mathcal{S}_\Omega(g) + \mathcal{D}_\Omega(U|_{\partial\Omega})$ in Ω by Green's formula, we have

$$\Big(\frac{1}{2}I - \mathcal{K}_\Omega\Big)(U|_{\partial\Omega}) = -(\mathcal{S}_\Omega g)|_{\partial\Omega} . \tag{3.42}$$

Since $\phi \in L_0^2(\partial D)$, it follows from (3.26) that

$$-\Big(\frac{1}{2}I - \mathcal{K}_\Omega\Big)((N_D \phi)|_{\partial\Omega}) = (\mathcal{S}_D \phi)|_{\partial\Omega} . \tag{3.43}$$

Then, from (3.41), (3.42), and (3.43), we conclude that

$$\Big(\frac{1}{2}I - \mathcal{K}_\Omega\Big)\Big(H|_{\partial\Omega} - U|_{\partial\Omega} + \Big(\frac{1}{2}I + \mathcal{K}_\Omega\Big)((N_D \phi)|_{\partial\Omega})\Big) = 0 .$$

Therefore, we have from Lemma 3.1.12

$$H|_{\partial\Omega} - U|_{\partial\Omega} + \Big(\frac{1}{2}I + \mathcal{K}_\Omega\Big)((N_D \phi)|_{\partial\Omega}) = C \text{ (constant)}. \tag{3.44}$$

Note from (3.28) that

$$(\frac{1}{2}I + \mathcal{K}_\Omega)((N_D \phi)|_{\partial\Omega}) = (N_D \phi)|_{\partial\Omega} + (\mathcal{S}_D \phi)|_{\partial\Omega} .$$

Thus we get from (3.33) and (3.44) that

$$u|_{\partial\Omega} = U|_{\partial\Omega} - (N_D \phi)|_{\partial\Omega} + C . \tag{3.45}$$

Since all the functions entering in (3.45) belong to $L_0^2(\partial\Omega)$, we conclude that $C = 0$, and the theorem is proved. $\square$

3.2 Helmholtz Equation

Consider the scalar wave equation $\partial_t^2 U - \Delta U = 0$. We obtain a time-harmonic solution $U(x,t) = \Re[e^{-i\omega t} u(x)]$ if the space-dependent part u satisfies the Helmholtz equation, $\Delta u + \omega^2 u = 0$.

Mathematical models for acoustical and microwave soundings of biological media involve the Helmholtz equation.

This section begins by discussing the well-known Sommerfeld radiation condition, and by deriving a fundamental solution. Next, we introduce the single- and double-layer potentials, and state Rellich's lemma. The final subsection establishes two decompositions formulae for the solution to the transmission problem.

3.2.1 Fundamental Solution

A fundamental solution $\Gamma_k(x)$ to the Helmholtz operator $\Delta + k^2$ in $\mathbb{R}^d$ is a solution (in the sense of distributions) of

$$(\Delta + k^2)\Gamma_k = \delta_0 \,, \tag{3.46}$$

where δ_0 is the Dirac mass at 0. Solutions are not unique, since we can add to a solution any plane wave (of the form $e^{ik\theta \cdot x}, \theta \in \mathbb{R}^d : |\theta| = 1$) or any combination of such plane waves. We need to specify the behavior of the solutions at infinity. It is natural to look for radial solutions of the form $\Gamma_k(x) = w_k(r)$ that is subject to the extra Sommerfeld radiation condition or outgoing wave condition

$$\left| \frac{dw_k}{dr} - ikw_k \right| \leq Cr^{-(d+1)/2} \quad \text{at infinity.} \tag{3.47}$$

If $d = 3$, equation (3.46) becomes

$$\frac{1}{r^2} \frac{d}{dr} r^2 \frac{dw_k}{dr} + k^2 w_k = 0, \quad r > 0 \,,$$

whose solution is

$$w_k(r) = c_1 \frac{e^{ikr}}{r} + c_2 \frac{e^{-ikr}}{r} \,.$$

It is easy to check that the Sommerfeld radiation condition (3.47) leads to $c_2 = 0$ and then (3.46) leads to $c_1 = -1/(4\pi)$.

If $d = 2$, equation (3.46) becomes

$$\frac{1}{r} \frac{d}{dr} r \frac{dw_k}{dr} + k^2 w_k = 0, \quad r > 0 \,.$$

This is a Bessel equation whose solutions are not elementary functions. From Sect. 2.1, we know that the Hankel functions of the first and second kind of order 0, $H_0^{(1)}(kr)$ and $H_0^{(2)}(kr)$, form a basis for the solution space. At infinity $(r \to +\infty)$, only $H_0^{(1)}(kr)$ satisfies the outgoing radiation condition (3.47). At the origin $(r \to 0)$, $H_0^{(1)}(kr)$ behaves like $(2i/\pi)\log(r)$. The following lemma holds.

Lemma 3.2.1 (Fundamental Solution) *The outgoing fundamental solution $\Gamma_k(x)$ to the operator $\Delta + k^2$ is given by*

$$\Gamma_k(x) = \begin{cases} -\dfrac{i}{4} H_0^{(1)}(k|x|) \,, & d = 2 \,, \\[2mm] -\dfrac{e^{ik|x|}}{4\pi|x|} \,, & d = 3 \,, \end{cases}$$

for $x \neq 0$, where $H_0^{(1)}$ is the Hankel function of the first kind of order 0.

Let for $x \neq 0$

$$\Gamma_0(x) := \Gamma(x) = \begin{cases} \dfrac{1}{2\pi} \log|x| \,, & d = 2 \,, \\[2mm] -\dfrac{1}{4\pi|x|} \,, & d = 3 \,. \end{cases}$$

3.2.2 Layer Potentials

For a bounded smooth domain D in $\mathbb{R}^d$ and $k > 0$ let $\mathcal{S}_D^k$ and $\mathcal{D}_D^k$ be the single- and double-layer potentials defined by Γ_k, that is,

$$\mathcal{S}_D^k \varphi(x) = \int_{\partial D} \Gamma_k(x-y)\varphi(y)\,d\sigma(y) \,, \quad x \in \mathbb{R}^d \,,$$

$$\mathcal{D}_D^k \varphi(x) = \int_{\partial D} \frac{\partial \Gamma_k(x-y)}{\partial \nu_y}\varphi(y)\,d\sigma(y) \,, \quad x \in \mathbb{R}^d \setminus \partial D \,,$$

for $\varphi \in L^2(\partial D)$. Because $\Gamma_k - \Gamma_0$ is a smooth function, we can easily prove from (3.20) and (3.17) that

$$\left.\frac{\partial(\mathcal{S}_D^k\varphi)}{\partial \nu}\right|_{\pm}(x) = \left(\pm\frac{1}{2}I + (\mathcal{K}_D^k)^*\right)\varphi(x) \quad \text{a.e. } x \in \partial D \,, \tag{3.48}$$

$$\left.(\mathcal{D}_D^k\varphi)\right|_{\pm}(x) = \left(\mp\frac{1}{2}I + \mathcal{K}_D^k\right)\varphi(x) \quad \text{a.e. } x \in \partial D \,, \tag{3.49}$$

for $\varphi \in L^2(\partial D)$, where $\mathcal{K}_D^k$ is the operator defined by

$$\mathcal{K}_D^k \varphi(x) = \int_{\partial D} \frac{\partial \Gamma_k(x-y)}{\partial \nu_y}\varphi(y)d\sigma(y) \,, \tag{3.50}$$

and $(\mathcal{K}_D^k)^*$ is the L^2-adjoint of $\mathcal{K}_D^{-k}$, that is,

$$(\mathcal{K}_D^k)^* \varphi(x) = \int_{\partial D} \frac{\partial \Gamma_k(x-y)}{\partial \nu_x} \varphi(y) d\sigma(y) \ . \tag{3.51}$$

Moreover, the integral operators $\mathcal{K}_D^k$ and $(\mathcal{K}_D^k)^*$ are compact on $L^2(\partial D)$.

We will need the following important result from the theory of the Helmholtz equation. It will help us to prove uniqueness for exterior Helmholtz problems. For its proof we refer to [44, Lemma 2.11] or [98, Lemma 9.8].

Lemma 3.2.2 (Rellich's Lemma) *Let $R_0 > 0$ and $B_R(0) = \{|x| < R\}$. Let u satisfy the Helmholtz equation $\Delta u + k^2 u = 0$ for $|x| > R_0$. Assume, furthermore, that*

$$\lim_{R \to +\infty} \int_{\partial B_R(0)} |u(x)|^2 \, d\sigma(x) = 0 \ .$$

Then, $u \equiv 0$ for $|x| > R_0$.

Note that the assertion of this lemma does not hold if k is imaginary or $k = 0$.

Now we can state the following uniqueness result for the Helmholtz equation.

Lemma 3.2.3 *Suppose $d = 2$ or 3. Let D be a bounded C^2-domain in $\mathbb{R}^d$. Let $u \in W_{\text{loc}}^{1,2}(\mathbb{R}^d \setminus \overline{D})$ satisfy*

$$\begin{cases} \Delta u + k^2 u = 0 & in \ \mathbb{R}^d \setminus \overline{D} \ , \\ \left| \dfrac{\partial u}{\partial r} - iku \right| = O\left(r^{-(d+1)/2} \right) & as \ r = |x| \to +\infty \quad uniformly \ in \ \dfrac{x}{|x|} \ , \\ \Im m \displaystyle\int_{\partial D} \overline{u} \dfrac{\partial u}{\partial \nu} \, d\sigma = 0 \ . \end{cases}$$

Then, $u \equiv 0$ in $\mathbb{R}^d \setminus \overline{D}$.

Proof. Let $B_R(0) = \{|x| < R\}$. For R large enough, $D \subset B_R(0)$. Notice first that by multiplying $\Delta u + k^2 u = 0$ by $\overline{u}$ and integrating by parts over $B_R(0) \setminus \overline{D}$ we arrive at

$$\Im m \int_{\partial B_R(0)} \overline{u} \frac{\partial u}{\partial \nu} \, d\sigma = 0 \ ,$$

since

$$\Im m \int_{\partial D} \overline{u} \frac{\partial u}{\partial \nu} \, d\sigma = 0 \ .$$

But

$$\Im m \int_{\partial B_R(0)} \overline{u} \left(\frac{\partial u}{\partial \nu} - iku \right) d\sigma = -k \int_{\partial B_R(0)} |u|^2 \ .$$

Applying the Cauchy–Schwarz inequality,

$$\left| \Im m \int_{\partial B_R(0)} \overline{u} \left(\frac{\partial u}{\partial \nu} - iku \right) d\sigma \right| \leq \left(\int_{\partial B_R(0)} |u|^2 \right)^{1/2} \left(\int_{\partial B_R(0)} \left| \frac{\partial u}{\partial \nu} - iku \right|^2 d\sigma \right)^{1/2}$$

and using the Sommerfeld radiation condition

$$\left| \frac{\partial u}{\partial r} - iku \right| = O\left(r^{-(d+1)/2} \right) \quad \text{as } r \to +\infty ,$$

we get

$$\left| \Im m \int_{\partial B_R(0)} \overline{u} \left(\frac{\partial u}{\partial \nu} - iku \right) d\sigma \right| \le \frac{C}{R} \left(\int_{\partial B_R(0)} |u|^2 \right)^{1/2} ,$$

for some positive constant C independent of R. Consequently, we obtain that

$$\left(\int_{\partial B_R(0)} |u|^2 \right)^{1/2} \le \frac{C}{R} ,$$

which indicates by Rellich's Lemma that $u \equiv 0$ in $\mathbb{R}^d \setminus \overline{B_R(0)}$. Hence, by the unique continuation property for $\Delta + k^2$, we can conclude that $u \equiv 0$ up to the boundary ∂D. This finishes the proof. $\square$

3.2.3 Transmission Problem

Introduce the piecewise-constant functions

$$\mu(x) = \begin{cases} \mu_0 , & x \in \Omega \setminus \overline{D} , \\ \mu_\star , & x \in D , \end{cases}$$

and

$$\varepsilon(x) = \begin{cases} \varepsilon_0 , & x \in \Omega \setminus \overline{D} , \\ \varepsilon_\star , & x \in D , \end{cases}$$

where $\mu_0, \mu_\star, \varepsilon_0,$ and $\varepsilon_\star$ are positive constants.

Let $f \in W_{\frac{1}{2}}^2(\partial \Omega)$, and let u and U denote the solutions to the Helmholtz equations

$$\begin{cases} \nabla \cdot \left(\frac{1}{\mu} \nabla u \right) + \omega^2 \varepsilon u = 0 \quad \text{in } \Omega , \\ u = f \quad \text{on } \partial \Omega , \end{cases} \tag{3.52}$$

and

$$\begin{cases} \Delta U + \omega^2 \varepsilon_0 \mu_0 U = 0 \quad \text{in } \Omega , \\ U = f \quad \text{on } \partial \Omega . \end{cases} \tag{3.53}$$

In electromagnetics, $\varepsilon_0, \varepsilon_\star$ are electrical permittivities, μ_0 and $\mu_\star$ are magnetic permeabilities, and u and U are electric fields. In acoustics, one replaces permittivity and permeability by compressibility and volume density of mass, and the scalar electric field by the scalar acoustic pressure.

We now present two decompositions of the solution of (3.52) similar to the representation formula (3.33) for the transmission problem for the harmonic equation. To do so, we first state the following theorem which is of importance to us for establishing our decomposition formulae. We refer the reader to [13] for its proof.

Theorem 3.2.4 *Let* $k_\star^2 := \omega^2 \mu_\star \varepsilon_\star$. *Suppose that* $k_0^2 := \omega^2 \mu_0 \varepsilon_0$ *is not a Dirichlet eigenvalue for* $-\Delta$ *on* D. *For each* $(F, G) \in W_1^2(\partial D) \times L^2(\partial D)$, *there exists a unique solution* $(f, g) \in L^2(\partial D) \times L^2(\partial D)$ *to the system of integral equations*

$$\begin{cases} \mathcal{S}_D^{k_\star} f - \mathcal{S}_D^{k_0} g = F \\ \dfrac{1}{\mu_\star} \dfrac{\partial(\mathcal{S}_D^{k_\star} f)}{\partial \nu}\bigg|_{-} - \dfrac{1}{\mu_0} \dfrac{\partial(\mathcal{S}_D^{k_0} g)}{\partial \nu}\bigg|_{+} = G \end{cases} \quad on \ \partial D . \qquad (3.54)$$

Furthermore, there exists a constant C *independent of* F *and* G *such that*

$$\|f\|_{L^2(\partial D)} + \|g\|_{L^2(\partial D)} \leq C \left(\|F\|_{W_1^2(\partial D)} + \|G\|_{L^2(\partial D)} \right) . \qquad (3.55)$$

The following decomposition formula holds.

Theorem 3.2.5 (Decomposition Formula) *Suppose that* k_0^2 *is not a Dirichlet eigenvalue for* $-\Delta$ *on* D. *Let* u *be the solution of (3.52) and* $g := \frac{\partial u}{\partial \nu}|_{\partial \Omega}$. *Define*

$$H(x) := -\mathcal{S}_\Omega^{k_0}(g)(x) + \mathcal{D}_\Omega^{k_0}(f)(x) , \quad x \in \mathbb{R}^d \setminus \partial \Omega , \qquad (3.56)$$

and let $(\varphi, \psi) \in L^2(\partial D) \times L^2(\partial D)$ *be the unique solution of*

$$\begin{cases} \mathcal{S}_D^{k_\star} \varphi - \mathcal{S}_D^{k_0} \psi = H \\ \dfrac{1}{\mu_\star} \dfrac{\partial(\mathcal{S}_D^{k_\star} \varphi)}{\partial \nu}\bigg|_{-} - \dfrac{1}{\mu_0} \dfrac{\partial(\mathcal{S}_D^{k_0} \psi)}{\partial \nu}\bigg|_{+} = \dfrac{1}{\mu_0} \dfrac{\partial H}{\partial \nu} \end{cases} \quad on \ \partial D . \qquad (3.57)$$

Then u *can be represented as*

$$u(x) = \begin{cases} H(x) + \mathcal{S}_D^{k_0} \psi(x) , & x \in \Omega \setminus \overline{D} , \\ \mathcal{S}_D^{k_\star} \varphi(x) , & x \in D . \end{cases} \qquad (3.58)$$

Moreover, there exists $C > 0$ *independent of* H *such that*

$$\|\varphi\|_{L^2(\partial D)} + \|\psi\|_{L^2(\partial D)} \leq C \left(\|H\|_{L^2(\partial D)} + \|\nabla H\|_{L^2(\partial D)} \right) . \qquad (3.59)$$

Proof. Note that u defined by (3.58) satisfies the differential equations and the transmission condition on ∂D in (3.52). Thus in order to prove (3.58), it suffices to prove that $\partial u/\partial \nu = g$ on $\partial \Omega$. Let $f := u|_{\partial \Omega}$ and consider the following transmission problem:

$$\begin{cases} (\Delta + k_0^2)v = 0 & \text{in } (\Omega \setminus \overline{D}) \cup (\mathbb{R}^d \setminus \overline{\Omega}) , \\ (\Delta + k_\star^2)v = 0 & \text{in } D , \\ v|_- - v|_+ = 0 , \quad \dfrac{1}{\mu_\star}\dfrac{\partial v}{\partial \nu}\Big|_- - \dfrac{1}{\mu_0}\dfrac{\partial v}{\partial \nu}\Big|_+ = 0 & \text{on } \partial D , \\ v|_- - v|_+ = f, \quad \dfrac{\partial v}{\partial \nu}\Big|_- - \dfrac{\partial v}{\partial \nu}\Big|_+ = g & \text{on } \partial \Omega , \\ \left|\dfrac{\partial v}{\partial r}(x) - ik_0 v(x)\right| = O(|x|^{-(d+1)/2}) , \quad |x| \to \infty . \end{cases} \tag{3.60}$$

We claim that (3.60) has a unique solution. In fact, if $f = g = 0$, then we can show as before that $v = 0$ in $\mathbb{R}^d \setminus \overline{D}$. Thus

$$v = \frac{\partial v}{\partial \nu}\Big|_- = 0 \quad \text{on } \partial D .$$

By the unique continuation for the operator $\Delta + k_\star^2$, we have $v = 0$ in D, and hence $v \equiv 0$ in $\mathbb{R}^d$. Note that v_p, $p = 1, 2$, defined by

$$v_1(x) = \begin{cases} u(x) , & x \in \Omega , \\ 0 , & x \in \mathbb{R}^d \setminus \overline{\Omega} , \end{cases} \qquad v_2(x) = \begin{cases} H(x) + \mathcal{S}_D^{k_0}\psi(x) , & x \in \Omega \setminus \overline{D} , \\ \mathcal{S}_D^{k_\star}\varphi(x) , & x \in D , \end{cases}$$

are two solutions of (3.60), and hence $v_1 \equiv v_2$. This completes the proof of solvability of (3.60). The estimate (3.59) is a consequence of solvability and the closed graph theorem. $\square$

The following proposition is also of importance to us. We refer again to [13] for a proof.

Proposition 3.2.6 *For each $n \in \mathbb{N}$ there exists C_n independent of D such that*

$$\|H\|_{\mathcal{C}^n(\overline{D})} \le C_n \|f\|_{W_{\frac{1}{2}}^2(\partial\Omega)} .$$

We now transform the decomposition formula (3.58) into the one using Green's function and the background solution U, that is, the solution of (3.53).

Let $G_{k_0}(x, y)$ be the Dirichlet Green function for $\Delta + k_0^2$ in Ω, *i.e.*, for each $y \in \Omega$, G is the solution of

$$\begin{cases} (\Delta + k_0^2)G_{k_0}(x, y) = \delta_y(x) , & x \in \Omega , \\ G_{k_0}(x, y) = 0 , & x \in \partial \Omega . \end{cases}$$

Then,

$$U(x) = \int_{\partial\Omega} \frac{\partial G_{k_0}(x, y)}{\partial \nu_y} f(y) d\sigma(y) , \quad x \in \Omega .$$

Introduce one more notation. For a $\mathcal{C}^2$-domain $D \subset\subset \Omega$ and $\varphi \in L^2(\partial D)$, let

$$G_D^{k_0}\varphi(x) := \int_{\partial D} G_{k_0}(x,y)\varphi(y)\,d\sigma(y)\,, \quad x \in \overline{\Omega}\,.$$

Our second decomposition formula is the following.

Theorem 3.2.7 *Let ψ be the function defined in (3.57). Then*

$$\frac{\partial u}{\partial \nu}(x) = \frac{\partial U}{\partial \nu}(x) + \frac{\partial(G_D^{k_0}\psi)}{\partial \nu}(x)\,, \quad x \in \partial\Omega\,. \tag{3.61}$$

To prove Theorem 3.2.7 we first observe an easy identity. If $x \in \mathbb{R}^d \setminus \Omega$ and $z \in \Omega$ then

$$\int_{\partial\Omega} \Gamma_{k_0}(x-y)\frac{\partial G_{k_0}(z,y)}{\partial \nu_y}\bigg|_{\partial\Omega} d\sigma(y) = \Gamma_{k_0}(x-z)\,. \tag{3.62}$$

As a consequence of (3.62), we have

$$\left(\frac{1}{2}I + (\mathcal{K}_\Omega^{k_0})^*\right)\left(\frac{\partial G_{k_0}(z,\cdot)}{\partial \nu_y}\bigg|_{\partial\Omega}\right)(x) = \frac{\partial \Gamma_{k_0}(x-z)}{\partial \nu_x}\,, \tag{3.63}$$

for all $x \in \partial\Omega$ and $z \in \Omega$.

Our second observation is the following.

Lemma 3.2.8 *If k_0^2 is not a Dirichlet eigenvalue for $-\Delta$ on Ω, then $(1/2)\,I + (\mathcal{K}_\Omega^{k_0})^* : L^2(\partial\Omega) \to L^2(\partial\Omega)$ is injective.*

Proof. Suppose that $\varphi \in L^2(\partial\Omega)$ and $\left((1/2)\,I + (\mathcal{K}_\Omega^{k_0})^*\right)\varphi = 0$. Define

$$u(x) := \mathcal{S}_\Omega^{k_0}\varphi(x)\,, x \in \mathbb{R}^d \setminus \overline{\Omega}\,.$$

Then u is a solution of $(\Delta + k_0^2)u = 0$ in $\mathbb{R}^d \setminus \overline{\Omega}$, and satisfies the Sommerfeld radiation condition

$$\left|\frac{\partial u}{\partial r} - ik_0 u\right| = O\left(r^{-(d+1)/2}\right) \quad \text{as } r \to +\infty\,,$$

and the Neumann boundary condition

$$\frac{\partial u}{\partial \nu}\bigg|_{\partial\Omega} = \left(\frac{1}{2}I + (\mathcal{K}_\Omega^{k_0})^*\right)\varphi = 0\,.$$

Therefore, by Lemma 3.2.3, we obtain $\mathcal{S}_\Omega^{k_0}\varphi(x) = 0$, $x \in \mathbb{R}^d \setminus \overline{\Omega}$. Since k_0^2 is not a Dirichlet eigenvalue for $-\Delta$ on Ω, we can prove that $\varphi \equiv 0$ in the same way as before. This completes the proof. $\square$

With these two observations available we are now ready to prove Theorem 3.2.7.

Proof of Theorem 3.2.7. Let $g := \partial u/\partial \nu$ and $g_0 := \partial U/\partial \nu$ on $\partial \Omega$ for convenience. By the divergence theorem, we get

$$U(x) = -\mathcal{S}_\Omega^{k_0}(g_0)(x) + \mathcal{D}_\Omega^{k_0}(f)(x) , \quad x \in \Omega .$$

It then follows from (3.56) that

$$H(x) = -\mathcal{S}_\Omega^{k_0}(g)(x) + \mathcal{S}_\Omega^{k_0}(g_0)(x) + U(x) , \quad x \in \Omega .$$

Consequently, substituting (3.58) into the above equation, we see that for $x \in \Omega$

$$H(x) = -\mathcal{S}_\Omega^{k_0}\left(\left.\frac{\partial H}{\partial \nu}\right|_{\partial \Omega} + \left.\frac{\partial(\mathcal{S}_D^{k_0}\psi)}{\partial \nu}\right|_{\partial \Omega}\right)(x) + \mathcal{S}_\Omega^{k_0}(g_0)(x) + U(x) .$$

Therefore the jump formula (3.48) yields

$$\frac{\partial H}{\partial \nu} = -\left(-\frac{1}{2}I + (\mathcal{K}_\Omega^{k_0})^* \right)\left(\left.\frac{\partial H}{\partial \nu}\right|_{\partial \Omega} + \left.\frac{\partial(\mathcal{S}_D^{k_0}\psi)}{\partial \nu}\right|_{\partial \Omega}\right)$$
$$+ \left(\frac{1}{2}I + (\mathcal{K}_\Omega^{k_0})^* \right)(g_0) \quad \text{on } \partial \Omega . \tag{3.64}$$

By (3.63), we have for $x \in \partial \Omega$

$$\frac{\partial(\mathcal{S}_D^{k_0}\psi)}{\partial \nu}(x) = \int_{\partial D} \frac{\partial \Gamma_{k_0}(x-y)}{\partial \nu_x}\psi(y)\,d\sigma(y)$$
$$= \left(\frac{1}{2}I + (\mathcal{K}_\Omega^{k_0})^* \right)\left(\left.\frac{\partial(G_D^{k_0}\psi)}{\partial \nu}\right|_{\partial \Omega}\right)(x) . \tag{3.65}$$

Thus we obtain

$$\left(-\frac{1}{2}I + (\mathcal{K}_\Omega^{k_0})^* \right)\left(\left.\frac{\partial(\mathcal{S}_D^{k_0}\psi)}{\partial \nu}\right|_{\partial \Omega}\right)$$
$$= \left(\frac{1}{2}I + (\mathcal{K}_\Omega^{k_0})^* \right)\left(\left(-\frac{1}{2}I + (\mathcal{K}_\Omega^{k_0})^* \right)\left(\left.\frac{\partial(G_D^{k_0}\psi)}{\partial \nu}\right|_{\partial \Omega}\right)\right) \quad \text{on } \partial \Omega .$$

It then follows from (3.64) that

$$\left(\frac{1}{2}I + (\mathcal{K}_\Omega^{k_0})^* \right)\left(\left.\frac{\partial H}{\partial \nu}\right|_{\partial \Omega} + \left(-\frac{1}{2}I + (\mathcal{K}_\Omega^{k_0})^* \right)\left(\left.\frac{\partial(G_D^{k_0}\psi)}{\partial \nu}\right|_{\partial \Omega}\right) - g_0 \right) = 0$$

on $\partial \Omega$ and hence, by Lemma 3.2.8, we arrive at

$$\left.\frac{\partial H}{\partial \nu}\right|_{\partial \Omega} + \left(-\frac{1}{2}I + (\mathcal{K}_\Omega^{k_0})^* \right)\left(\left.\frac{\partial(G_D^{k_0}\psi)}{\partial \nu}\right|_{\partial \Omega}\right) - g_0 = 0 \quad \text{on } \partial \Omega . \tag{3.66}$$

By substituting this equation into (3.58), we get

$$\frac{\partial u}{\partial \nu} = \frac{\partial U}{\partial \nu} - \left(-\frac{1}{2}I + (\mathcal{K}_\Omega^{k_0})^* \right) \left(\frac{\partial (G_D^{k_0} \psi)}{\partial \nu} \bigg|_{\partial \Omega} \right) + \frac{\partial (\mathcal{S}_D^{k_0} \psi)}{\partial \nu} \quad \text{on } \partial \Omega .$$

Finally, using (3.65) we conclude that (3.61) holds and the proof is then complete. □

Observe that, by (3.48), (3.66) is equivalent to

$$\frac{\partial}{\partial \nu} \left(H + \mathcal{S}_\Omega^{k_0} \left(\frac{\partial (G_D^{k_0} \psi)}{\partial \nu} \bigg|_{\partial \Omega} \right) - U \right) \bigg|_- = 0 \quad \text{on } \partial \Omega .$$

On the other hand, by (3.62),

$$\mathcal{S}_\Omega^{k_0} \left(\frac{\partial (G_D^{k_0} \psi)}{\partial \nu} \bigg|_{\partial \Omega} \right)(x) = \mathcal{S}_D^{k_0} \psi(x) , \quad x \in \partial \Omega .$$

Thus, by (3.58), we obtain

$$H(x) + \mathcal{S}_\Omega^{k_0} \left(\frac{\partial (G_D^{k_0} \psi)}{\partial \nu} \bigg|_{\partial \Omega} \right)(x) - U(x) = 0 , \quad x \in \partial \Omega .$$

Then, by the unique continuation for $\Delta + k_0^2$, we obtain the following Lemma.

Lemma 3.2.9 *We have*

$$H(x) = U(x) - \mathcal{S}_\Omega^{k_0} \left(\frac{\partial (G_D^{k_0} \psi)}{\partial \nu} \bigg|_{\partial \Omega} \right)(x) , \quad x \in \Omega . \tag{3.67}$$

3.3 Static Elasticity

In the preceding two sections, we considered the simplest and most important examples of scalar elliptic equations. Now we turn to the best-known example of an elliptic system, namely, the Lamé system.

This section begins with a derivation of the standard two- and three-dimensional fundamental solutions. After that, we introduce the single- and double-layer potentials and state their jump relations and their mapping properties. Extra difficulties in solving the elasticity system using a layer potential technique come from the fact that the corresponding integral operators to $\mathcal{K}_D$ and $\mathcal{K}_D^*$, that arise when studying Laplace's equation, are not compact. We also have to handle carefully the fact that the Neumann problem in linear elasticity has a (finite-dimensional) kernel. The final subsection investigates the transmission problem. A decomposition formula for the displacement field, analogous to those established in the two previous subsections, is derived.

3.3.1 Fundamental Solution

Let D be a bounded smooth domain in $\mathbb{R}^d$, $d = 2, 3$, and (λ, μ) be the Lamé constants for D satisfying

$$\mu > 0 \quad \text{and} \quad d\lambda + 2\mu > 0 \,.$$

See Kupradze [85]. The constants λ and μ are respectively referred to as the compression modulus and the shear modulus.

In a homogeneous elastic medium, the elastostatic system corresponding to the Lamé constants λ, μ is defined by

$$\mathcal{L}_{\lambda,\mu}\mathbf{u} := \mu \Delta \mathbf{u} + (\lambda + \mu)\nabla\nabla \cdot \mathbf{u} \,.$$

The corresponding conormal derivative $\partial \mathbf{u}/\partial \nu$ on ∂D is defined to be

$$\frac{\partial \mathbf{u}}{\partial \nu} := \lambda(\nabla \cdot \mathbf{u})N + \mu(\nabla \mathbf{u} + \nabla \mathbf{u}^T)N \quad \text{on } \partial D \,, \tag{3.68}$$

where N is the outward unit normal to ∂D and the superscript T denotes the transpose of a matrix.

Notice that the conormal derivative has a direct physical meaning:

$$\frac{\partial \mathbf{u}}{\partial \nu} = \text{traction on } \partial D \,.$$

The vector $\mathbf{u}$ is the displacement field of the elastic medium having the Lamé coefficients λ and μ, and $(\nabla \mathbf{u} + \nabla \mathbf{u}^T)/2$ is the strain tensor.

Let us state a simple, but important relation. The identity (3.69) is referred to as the divergence theorem.

Lemma 3.3.1 *If* $\mathbf{u} \in W^{1,2}(D)$ *and* $\mathcal{L}_{\lambda,\mu}\mathbf{u} = 0$ *in* D, *then for all* $\mathbf{v} \in W^{1,2}(D)$,

$$\int_{\partial D} \mathbf{v} \cdot \frac{\partial \mathbf{u}}{\partial \nu}\, d\sigma = \int_D \lambda(\nabla \cdot \mathbf{u})(\nabla \cdot \mathbf{v}) + \frac{\mu}{2}(\nabla \mathbf{u} + \nabla \mathbf{u}^T) \cdot (\nabla \mathbf{v} + \nabla \mathbf{v}^T)\, dx \,, \tag{3.69}$$

where for $d \times d$ *matrices* $a = (a_{ij})$ *and* $b = (b_{ij})$, $a \cdot b = \sum_{ij} a_{ij} b_{ij}$.

Proof.   By the definition (3.68) of the conormal derivative, we get

$$\int_{\partial D} \mathbf{v} \cdot \frac{\partial \mathbf{u}}{\partial \nu}\, d\sigma = \int_{\partial D} \lambda(\nabla \cdot \mathbf{u})\mathbf{v} \cdot N + \mu \mathbf{v} \cdot (\nabla \mathbf{u} + \nabla \mathbf{u}^T)N\, d\sigma$$

$$= \int_D \lambda \nabla \cdot ((\nabla \cdot \mathbf{u})\mathbf{v}) + \mu \nabla \cdot ((\nabla \mathbf{u} + \nabla \mathbf{u}^T)\mathbf{v})\, dx \,.$$

Since

$$\nabla \cdot \left((\nabla \mathbf{u} + \nabla \mathbf{u}^T)\mathbf{v} \right) = \nabla(\nabla \cdot \mathbf{u}) \cdot \mathbf{v} + \Delta \mathbf{u} \cdot \mathbf{v} + \frac{1}{2}(\nabla \mathbf{u} + \nabla \mathbf{u}^T) \cdot (\nabla \mathbf{v} + \nabla \mathbf{v}^T) \,,$$

we obtain (3.69) and the proof is complete. $\square$

We give now a fundamental solution to the Lamé system $\mathcal{L}_{\lambda,\mu}$ in $\mathbb{R}^d$.

Lemma 3.3.2 (Fundamental Solution) *A fundamental solution* $\Gamma = (\Gamma_{ij})_{i,j=1}^d$ *to the Lamé system* $\mathcal{L}_{\lambda,\mu}$ *is given by*

$$
\Gamma_{ij}(x) := \begin{cases}
-\dfrac{A}{4\pi}\dfrac{\delta_{ij}}{|x|} - \dfrac{B}{4\pi}\dfrac{x_i x_j}{|x|^3} & \text{if } d = 3\,, \\[2ex]
\dfrac{A}{2\pi}\delta_{ij}\ln|x| - \dfrac{B}{2\pi}\dfrac{x_i x_j}{|x|^2} & \text{if } d = 2\,,
\end{cases} \qquad x \neq 0\,, \qquad (3.70)
$$

where

$$
A = \frac{1}{2}\left(\frac{1}{\mu} + \frac{1}{2\mu+\lambda}\right) \quad \text{and} \quad B = \frac{1}{2}\left(\frac{1}{\mu} - \frac{1}{2\mu+\lambda}\right)\,. \qquad (3.71)
$$

The function Γ *is known as the Kelvin matrix of fundamental solutions.*

Proof. We seek a solution $\Gamma = (\Gamma_{ij})_{i,j=1}^d$ of

$$
\mu\Delta\Gamma + (\lambda + \mu)\nabla\nabla\cdot\Gamma = \delta_0 I_d \quad \text{in } \mathbb{R}^d\,, \qquad (3.72)
$$

where I_d is the $d \times d$ identity matrix and δ_0 is the Dirac mass at 0.

Taking the divergence of (3.72), we have

$$
(\lambda + 2\mu)\Delta(\nabla\cdot\Gamma) = \nabla\delta_0\,.
$$

Thus by Lemma 3.1.1

$$
\nabla\cdot\Gamma = \frac{1}{\lambda + 2\mu}\nabla\Gamma\,,
$$

where Γ is given by (3.1). Inserting this into (3.72) gives

$$
\mu\Delta\Gamma = \delta_0 I_d - \frac{\lambda + \mu}{\lambda + 2\mu}\nabla\nabla\Gamma\,.
$$

Hence it follows that

$$
\Gamma_{ij}(x) := \begin{cases}
-\dfrac{A}{4\pi}\dfrac{\delta_{ij}}{|x|} - \dfrac{B}{4\pi}\dfrac{x_i x_j}{|x|^3} & \text{if } d = 3\,, \\[2ex]
\dfrac{A}{2\pi}\delta_{ij}\ln|x| - \dfrac{B}{2\pi}\dfrac{x_i x_j}{|x|^2} & \text{if } d = 2\,,
\end{cases} \qquad x \neq 0\,,
$$

modulo constants, where A and B are given by (3.71). $\square$

We refer to McLean [98, Theorem 10.4] for an alternative approach for obtaining a fundamental solution for the elasticity operator.

3.3.2 Layer Potentials

The single- and double-layer potentials of the density function φ on D associated with the Lamé parameters (λ, μ) are defined by

$$\mathcal{S}_D\varphi(x) := \int_{\partial D} \Gamma(x - y)\varphi(y)\, d\sigma(y)\ , \quad x \in \mathbb{R}^d\ , \tag{3.73}$$

$$\mathcal{D}_D\varphi(x) := \int_{\partial D} \frac{\partial}{\partial \nu_y}\Gamma(x - y)\varphi(y)\, d\sigma(y)\ , \quad x \in \mathbb{R}^d \setminus \partial D\ , \tag{3.74}$$

where $\partial/\partial\nu$ denotes the conormal derivative defined in (3.68). Thus, for $m = 1, \ldots, d$,

$$(\mathcal{D}_D\varphi(x))_m = \int_{\partial D} \lambda\frac{\partial \Gamma_{mi}}{\partial y_i}(x - y)\varphi(y) \cdot N(y)$$
$$+ \mu\left(\frac{\partial \Gamma_{mi}}{\partial y_j} + \frac{\partial \Gamma_{mj}}{\partial y_i}\right)(x - y)N_i(y)\varphi_j(y)\, d\sigma(y)\ .$$

Here we used the Einstein convention for the summation notation. As an immediate consequence of (3.69) we obtain the following lemma which can be proved in the same way as the Green representation (3.4) of harmonic functions.

Lemma 3.3.3 *If* $\mathbf{u} \in W^{1,2}(D)$ *and* $\mathcal{L}_{\lambda,\mu}\mathbf{u} = 0$ *in* D, *then*

$$\mathbf{u}(x) = \mathcal{D}_D(\mathbf{u}|_{\partial D})(x) - \mathcal{S}_D\left(\frac{\partial \mathbf{u}}{\partial \nu}\bigg|_{\partial D}\right)(x)\ , \quad x \in D\ , \tag{3.75}$$

and

$$\mathcal{D}_D(\mathbf{u}|_{\partial D})(x) - \mathcal{S}_D\left(\frac{\partial \mathbf{u}}{\partial \nu}\bigg|_{\partial D}\right)(x) = 0\ , \quad x \in \mathbb{R}^d \setminus \overline{D}\ . \tag{3.76}$$

As before, let $\mathbf{u}|_+$ and $\mathbf{u}|_-$ denote the limits from outside D and inside D, respectively.

Theorem 3.3.4 (Trace Formulae) *Let* D *be a bounded smooth domain in* $\mathbb{R}^d, d = 2$ *or* 3. *For* $\varphi \in L^2(\partial D)$

$$\mathcal{D}_D\varphi|_\pm = (\mp\frac{1}{2}I + \mathcal{K}_D)\varphi \quad a.e.\ on\ \partial D\ , \tag{3.77}$$

$$\frac{\partial}{\partial \nu}\mathcal{S}_D\varphi\Big|_\pm = (\pm\frac{1}{2}I + \mathcal{K}_D^*)\varphi \quad a.e.\ on\ \partial D\ , \tag{3.78}$$

where $\mathcal{K}_D$ *is defined by*

$$\mathcal{K}_D\varphi(x) := p.v. \int_{\partial D} \frac{\partial}{\partial \nu_y}\Gamma(x - y)\varphi(y)\, d\sigma(y) \quad a.e.\ x \in \partial D\ ,$$

and $\mathcal{K}_D^*$ *is the adjoint operator of* $\mathcal{K}_D$ *on* $L^2(\partial D)$, *i.e.,*

$$\mathcal{K}_D^*\varphi(x) := \text{p.v.} \int_{\partial D} \frac{\partial}{\partial \nu_x} \Gamma(x-y)\varphi(y)\, d\sigma(y) \quad a.e. \ x \in \partial D .$$

Here p.v. denotes the Cauchy principal value.

It must be emphasized once again that, in contrast with the corresponding integral operators that arise when studying Laplace's equation, the singular integral operator $\mathcal{K}_D$ is not compact. This causes some extra difficulties in solving the elasticity system using a layer potential technique.

We now determine all solutions of the homogeneous Neumann problem. Let Ψ be the vector space of all linear solutions of the equation $\mathcal{L}_{\lambda,\mu}\mathbf{u} = 0$ and $\partial\mathbf{u}/\partial\nu = 0$ on ∂D, or alternatively,

$$\Psi := \left\{ \psi : \partial_i \psi_j + \partial_j \psi_i = 0, \quad 1 \le i, j \le d \right\}. \tag{3.79}$$

Here ψ_i for $i = 1, \dots, d$, denote the components of ψ.

Observe now that the space Ψ is defined independently of the Lamé constants λ, μ and its dimension is 3 if $d = 2$ and 6 if $d = 3$. Define

$$L_\Psi^2(\partial D) := \left\{ \mathbf{f} \in L^2(\partial D) : \int_{\partial D} \mathbf{f} \cdot \psi\, d\sigma = 0 \text{ for all } \psi \in \Psi \right\} \tag{3.80}$$

a subspace of codimension $d(d+1)/2$ in $L^2(\partial D)$.

In particular, since Ψ contains constant functions, we get

$$\int_{\partial D} \mathbf{f}\, d\sigma = 0$$

for any $\mathbf{f} \in L_\Psi^2(\partial D)$. The following fact, which immediately follows from (3.69), is useful in later sections.

If $\mathbf{u} \in W^{1,\frac{3}{2}}(D)$ satisfies $\mathcal{L}_{\lambda,\mu}\mathbf{u} = 0$ in D, then $\left.\dfrac{\partial\mathbf{u}}{\partial\nu}\right|_{\partial D} \in L_\Psi^2(\partial D).$ $\quad$ (3.81)

One of fundamental results in the theory of linear elasticity using layer potentials is the following invertibility result.

Theorem 3.3.5 *The operator $\mathcal{K}_D$ is bounded on $L^2(\partial D)$, and $-(1/2)\,I + \mathcal{K}_D^*$ and $(1/2)\,I + \mathcal{K}_D^*$ are invertible on $L_\Psi^2(\partial D)$ and $L^2(\partial D)$, respectively.*

As a consequence of (3.78), we are able to state the following.

Corollary 3.3.6 *For a given $\mathbf{g} \in L_\Psi^2(\partial D)$, the function $\mathbf{u} \in W^{1,2}(D)$ defined by*

$$\mathbf{u}(x) := \mathcal{S}_D(-\frac{1}{2}I + \mathcal{K}_D^*)^{-1}\mathbf{g} \tag{3.82}$$

is a solution to the problem

$$\begin{cases} \mathcal{L}_{\lambda,\mu}\mathbf{u} = 0 & in \ D , \\ \left.\dfrac{\partial\mathbf{u}}{\partial\nu}\right|_{\partial D} = \mathbf{g} , & (\mathbf{u}|_{\partial D} \in L_\Psi^2(\partial D)) . \end{cases} \tag{3.83}$$

If $\psi \in \Psi$ and $x \in \mathbb{R}^d \setminus \overline{D}$, then from (3.69) it follows that $\mathcal{D}_D \psi(x) = 0$. Hence by (3.77), ψ satisfies $(-(1/2)\, I + \mathcal{K}_D)\psi = 0$. Since the dimension of the orthogonal complement of the range of the operator $-(1/2)\, I + \mathcal{K}_D^*$ is less than 3 if $d = 2$ and 6 if $d = 3$, which is the dimension of the space Ψ, we obtain the following corollary.

Corollary 3.3.7 *The null space of* $-(1/2)\, I + \mathcal{K}_D$ *on* $L^2(\partial D)$ *is* Ψ.

3.3.3 Transmission Problem

We suppose that the elastic medium Ω contains a single anomaly D which is also a bounded $\mathcal{C}^2$-domain. Let the constants (λ, μ) denote the background Lamé coefficients that are the elastic parameters in the absence of any anomalies. Suppose that D has a pair of Lamé constants $(\widetilde{\lambda}, \widetilde{\mu})$ which is different from that of the background elastic body, (λ, μ). It is always assumed that

$$\mu > 0, \quad d\lambda + 2\mu > 0, \quad \widetilde{\mu} > 0, \quad \text{and} \quad d\widetilde{\lambda} + 2\widetilde{\mu} > 0 . \tag{3.84}$$

We also assume that

$$(\lambda - \widetilde{\lambda})(\mu - \widetilde{\mu}) \geq 0, \quad \left((\lambda - \widetilde{\lambda})^2 + (\mu - \widetilde{\mu})^2 \neq 0\right) . \tag{3.85}$$

We consider the transmission problem

$$\begin{cases} \displaystyle\sum_{j,k,l=1}^{d} \frac{\partial}{\partial x_j}\left(C_{ijkl}\frac{\partial u_k}{\partial x_l}\right) = 0 \quad \text{in } \Omega, \quad i = 1,\dots,d , \\[2mm] \left.\dfrac{\partial \mathbf{u}}{\partial \nu}\right|_{\partial \Omega} = \mathbf{g} , \end{cases} \tag{3.86}$$

where the elasticity tensor $C = (C_{ijkl})$ is given by

$$\begin{aligned} C_{ijkl} := {}&\left(\lambda\,\chi(\Omega \setminus D) + \widetilde{\lambda}\,\chi(D)\right)\delta_{ij}\delta_{kl} \\ &+\left(\mu\,\chi(\Omega \setminus D) + \widetilde{\mu}\,\chi(D)\right)(\delta_{ik}\delta_{jl} + \delta_{il}\delta_{jk}) , \end{aligned} \tag{3.87}$$

and u_k for $k = 1,\dots,d$, denote the components of the displacement field $\mathbf{u}$.

In order to ensure existence and uniqueness of a solution to (3.86), we assume that $\mathbf{g} \in L^2_\Psi(\partial \Omega)$ and seek a solution $\mathbf{u} \in W^{1,2}(\Omega)$ such that $\mathbf{u}|_{\partial \Omega} \in L^2_\Psi(\partial \Omega)$. The problem (3.86) is understood in a weak sense, namely, for any $\varphi \in W^{1,2}(\Omega)$ the following equality holds:

$$\sum_{i,j,k,l=1}^{d} \int_\Omega C_{ijkl}\frac{\partial u_k}{\partial x_l}\frac{\partial \varphi_i}{\partial x_j}\,dx = \int_{\partial \Omega} \mathbf{g} \cdot \varphi\,d\sigma ,$$

where φ_i for $i = 1,\dots,d$, denote the components of φ.

Let $\mathcal{L}_{\tilde{\lambda},\tilde{\mu}}$ and $\partial/\partial\tilde{\nu}$ be the Lamé system and the conormal derivative associated with $(\tilde{\lambda},\tilde{\mu})$, respectively. Then, for any $\varphi \in \mathcal{C}_0^\infty(\Omega)$, we compute

$$0 = \sum_{i,j,k,l=1}^{d} \int_\Omega C_{ijkl} \frac{\partial u_k}{\partial x_l} \frac{\partial \varphi_i}{\partial x_j} \, dx$$

$$= \int_{\Omega\setminus\overline{D}} \lambda(\nabla \cdot \mathbf{u})(\nabla \cdot \varphi) + \frac{\mu}{2}(\nabla\mathbf{u} + \nabla\mathbf{u}^T) \cdot (\nabla\varphi + \nabla\varphi^T) \, dx$$

$$+ \int_D \tilde{\lambda}(\nabla \cdot \mathbf{u})(\nabla \cdot \varphi) + \frac{\tilde{\mu}}{2}(\nabla\mathbf{u} + \nabla\mathbf{u}^T) \cdot (\nabla\varphi + \nabla\varphi^T) \, dx$$

$$= -\int_{\Omega\setminus\overline{D}} \mathcal{L}_{\lambda,\mu}\mathbf{u} \cdot \varphi \, dx - \int_{\partial D} \frac{\partial\mathbf{u}}{\partial\nu} \cdot \varphi \, d\sigma - \int_D \mathcal{L}_{\tilde{\lambda},\tilde{\mu}}\mathbf{u} \cdot \varphi \, dx + \int_{\partial D} \frac{\partial\mathbf{u}}{\partial\tilde{\nu}} \cdot \varphi \, d\sigma \,,$$

where the last equality follows from (3.69). Thus (3.86) is equivalent to the following problem:

$$\begin{cases} \mathcal{L}_{\lambda,\mu}\mathbf{u} = 0 & \text{in } \Omega\setminus\overline{D}\,, \\ \mathcal{L}_{\tilde{\lambda},\tilde{\mu}}\mathbf{u} = 0 & \text{in } D\,, \\ \mathbf{u}\big|_- = \mathbf{u}\big|_+ & \text{on } \partial D\,, \\ \dfrac{\partial\mathbf{u}}{\partial\tilde{\nu}}\bigg|_- = \dfrac{\partial\mathbf{u}}{\partial\nu}\bigg|_+ & \text{on } \partial D\,, \\ \dfrac{\partial\mathbf{u}}{\partial\nu}\bigg|_{\partial\Omega} = \mathbf{g}\,, & \left(\mathbf{u}|_{\partial\Omega} \in L_\Psi^2(\partial\Omega)\right). \end{cases} \qquad (3.88)$$

We denote by $\mathcal{S}_D$ and $\tilde{\mathcal{S}}_D$ the single layer potentials on ∂D corresponding to the Lamé constants (λ,μ) and $(\tilde{\lambda},\tilde{\mu})$, respectively. Suppose that

$$\partial D = \left\{ (\tilde{x}, x_d) : x_d = \varphi(\tilde{x}) \right\}.$$

We refer to $\|\nabla\varphi\|_{L^\infty(\mathbb{R}^{d-1})}$ as the Lipschitz-character of D.

The following result holds.

Theorem 3.3.8 *Suppose that* $(\lambda - \tilde{\lambda})(\mu - \tilde{\mu}) \geq 0$ *and* $0 < \tilde{\lambda}, \tilde{\mu} < +\infty$. *For any given* $(\mathbf{F}, \mathbf{G}) \in W_1^2(\partial D) \times L^2(\partial D)$, *there exists a unique pair* $(\mathbf{f}, \mathbf{g}) \in L^2(\partial D) \times L^2(\partial D)$ *such that*

$$\begin{cases} \tilde{\mathcal{S}}_D\mathbf{f}\big|_- - \mathcal{S}_D\mathbf{g}\big|_+ = \mathbf{F} & \text{on } \partial D\,, \\ \dfrac{\partial}{\partial\tilde{\nu}}\tilde{\mathcal{S}}_D\mathbf{f}\bigg|_- - \dfrac{\partial}{\partial\nu}\mathcal{S}_D\mathbf{g}\bigg|_+ = \mathbf{G} & \text{on } \partial D\,, \end{cases} \qquad (3.89)$$

and there exists a constant C *depending only on* λ, μ, $\tilde{\lambda}$, $\tilde{\mu}$, *and the Lipschitz-character of* D *such that*

$$\|\mathbf{f}\|_{L^2(\partial D)} + \|\mathbf{g}\|_{L^2(\partial D)} \le C\left(\|\mathbf{F}\|_{W_1^2(\partial D)} + \|\mathbf{G}\|_{L^2(\partial D)}\right) . \tag{3.90}$$

Moreover, if $\mathbf{G} \in L_\Psi^2(\partial D)$, *then* $\mathbf{g} \in L_\Psi^2(\partial D)$.

Proof. The proof of the unique solvability of the integral equation (3.89) is omitted. By (3.81), $\partial \widetilde{\mathcal{S}}_D \mathbf{f}/\partial \tilde{\nu}|_- \in L_\Psi^2(\partial D)$. Thus if $\mathbf{G} \in L_\Psi^2(\partial D)$, then $\partial \mathcal{S}_D \mathbf{g}/\partial \nu|_+ \in L_\Psi^2(\partial D)$. Since

$$\mathbf{g} = \left.\frac{\partial}{\partial \nu}\mathcal{S}_D \mathbf{g}\right|_+ - \left.\frac{\partial}{\partial \nu}\mathcal{S}_D \mathbf{g}\right|_- ,$$

then, by (3.78) and $\partial \mathcal{S}_D \mathbf{g}/\partial \nu|_- \in L_\Psi^2(\partial D)$, we conclude that $\mathbf{g} \in L_\Psi^2(\partial D)$. $\square$

Lemma 3.3.9 *Let* $\varphi \in \Psi$. *If the pair* $(\mathbf{f}, \mathbf{g}) \in L^2(\partial D) \times L_\Psi^2(\partial D)$ *is the solution of*

$$\begin{cases} \left.\widetilde{\mathcal{S}}_D \mathbf{f}\right|_- - \left.\mathcal{S}_D \mathbf{g}\right|_+ = \varphi|_{\partial D} , \\ \left.\dfrac{\partial}{\partial \tilde{\nu}}\widetilde{\mathcal{S}}_D \mathbf{f}\right|_- - \left.\dfrac{\partial}{\partial \nu}\mathcal{S}_D \mathbf{g}\right|_+ = 0 , \end{cases} \tag{3.91}$$

then $\mathbf{g} = 0$.

Proof. Define $\mathbf{u}$ by

$$\mathbf{u}(x) := \begin{cases} \mathcal{S}_D \mathbf{g}(x) , & x \in \mathbb{R}^d \setminus \overline{D} , \\ \widetilde{\mathcal{S}}_D \mathbf{f}(x) - \varphi(x) , & x \in D . \end{cases}$$

Since $\mathbf{g} \in L_\Psi^2(\partial D)$, then $\int_{\partial D} \mathbf{g}\, d\sigma = 0$, and hence

$$\mathcal{S}_D \mathbf{g}(x) = O(|x|^{1-d}) \quad \text{as } |x| \to +\infty .$$

Therefore $\mathbf{u}$ is the unique solution of

$$\begin{cases} \mathcal{L}_{\lambda,\mu}\mathbf{u} = 0 & \text{in } \mathbb{R}^d \setminus \overline{D} , \\ \mathcal{L}_{\tilde{\lambda},\tilde{\mu}}\mathbf{u} = 0 & \text{in } D , \\ \mathbf{u}|_+ = \mathbf{u}|_- & \text{on } \partial D , \\ \left.\dfrac{\partial \mathbf{u}}{\partial \nu}\right|_+ = \left.\dfrac{\partial \mathbf{u}}{\partial \tilde{\nu}}\right|_- & \text{on } \partial D , \\ \mathbf{u}(x) = O(|x|^{1-d}) & \text{as } |x| \to +\infty . \end{cases} \tag{3.92}$$

Using the fact that the trivial solution is the unique solution to (3.92), we see that

$$\mathcal{S}_D \mathbf{g}(x) = 0 \quad \text{for } x \in \mathbb{R}^d \setminus \overline{D} .$$

It then follows that $\mathcal{L}_{\lambda,\mu}\mathcal{S}_D\mathbf{g}(x) = 0$ for $x \in D$ and $\mathcal{S}_D\mathbf{g}(x) = 0$ for $x \in \partial D$. Thus, $\mathcal{S}_D\mathbf{g}(x) = 0$ for $x \in D$. Since

$$\mathbf{g} = \left.\frac{\partial(\mathcal{S}_D\mathbf{g})}{\partial \nu}\right|_+ - \left.\frac{\partial(\mathcal{S}_D\mathbf{g})}{\partial \nu}\right|_- ,$$

it is obvious that $\mathbf{g} = 0$.   □

We now state a decomposition theorem for the solution of the transmission problem. Again, we refer to [13] for its proof.

Theorem 3.3.10 (Decomposition Formula) *There exists a unique pair* $(\varphi, \psi) \in L^2(\partial D) \times L^2_{\Psi}(\partial D)$ *such that the solution* $\mathbf{u}$ *of (3.88) is represented by*

$$\mathbf{u}(x) = \begin{cases} \mathbf{H}(x) + \mathcal{S}_D\psi(x) , & x \in \Omega \setminus \overline{D} , \\ \widetilde{\mathcal{S}}_D\varphi(x) , & x \in D , \end{cases} \qquad (3.93)$$

where $\mathbf{H}$ *is defined by*

$$\mathbf{H}(x) = \mathcal{D}_\Omega(\mathbf{u}|_{\partial\Omega})(x) - \mathcal{S}_\Omega(\mathbf{g})(x) , \qquad x \in \mathbb{R}^d \setminus \partial\Omega . \qquad (3.94)$$

In fact, the pair (φ, ψ) *is the unique solution in* $L^2(\partial D) \times L^2_{\Psi}(\partial D)$ *of*

$$\begin{cases} \left.\widetilde{\mathcal{S}}_D\varphi\right|_- - \left.\mathcal{S}_D\psi\right|_+ = \mathbf{H}|_{\partial D} & on \ \partial D , \\ \left.\frac{\partial}{\partial\tilde{\nu}}\widetilde{\mathcal{S}}_D\varphi\right|_- - \left.\frac{\partial}{\partial\nu}\mathcal{S}_D\psi\right|_+ = \left.\frac{\partial\mathbf{H}}{\partial\nu}\right|_{\partial D} & on \ \partial D . \end{cases} \qquad (3.95)$$

There exists a positive constant C *such that*

$$\|\varphi\|_{L^2(\partial D)} + \|\psi\|_{L^2(\partial D)} \leq C\|\mathbf{H}\|_{W^2_1(\partial D)} . \qquad (3.96)$$

For any integer n, *there exists a positive constant* C_n *depending only on* c_0 *and* λ, μ *(not on* $\tilde{\lambda}, \tilde{\mu}$*) such that*

$$\|\mathbf{H}\|_{\mathcal{C}^n(\overline{D})} \leq C_n\|\mathbf{g}\|_{L^2(\partial\Omega)} . \qquad (3.97)$$

Moreover,

$$\mathbf{H}(x) = -\mathcal{S}_D\psi(x) , \qquad x \in \mathbb{R}^d \setminus \overline{\Omega} . \qquad (3.98)$$

We now derive a representation for $\mathbf{u}$ in terms of the background solution. Let $\mathbf{N}(x, y)$ be the Neumann function for $\mathcal{L}_{\lambda,\mu}$ in Ω corresponding to a Dirac mass at y. That is, $\mathbf{N}$ is the solution to

$$\begin{cases} \mathcal{L}_{\lambda,\mu}\mathbf{N}(x, y) = -\delta_y(x)I_d & in \ \Omega, \\ \left.\frac{\partial\mathbf{N}}{\partial\nu}\right|_{\partial\Omega} = -\frac{1}{|\partial\Omega|}I_d , \\ \mathbf{N}(\cdot, y) \in L^2_{\Psi}(\partial\Omega) & for \ any \ y \in \Omega , \end{cases} \qquad (3.99)$$

where the differentiations act on the x-variables, and I_d is the $d \times d$ identity matrix.

For $\mathbf{g} \in L^2_\psi(\partial\Omega)$, define

$$\mathbf{U}(x) := \int_{\partial\Omega} \mathbf{N}(x,y)\mathbf{g}(y)\, d\sigma(y) , \quad x \in \Omega . \tag{3.100}$$

Then $\mathbf{U}$ is the solution to (3.83) with D replaced by Ω. On the other hand, by (3.82), the solution to (3.83) is given by

$$\mathbf{U}(x) := \mathcal{S}_\Omega \left(-\frac{1}{2}I + \mathcal{K}^*_\Omega \right)^{-1} \mathbf{g}(x) .$$

Thus,

$$\int_{\partial\Omega} \mathbf{N}(x,y)\mathbf{g}(y)\, d\sigma(y) = \int_{\partial\Omega} \mathbf{\Gamma}(x-y)(-\frac{1}{2}I + \mathcal{K}^*_\Omega)^{-1}\mathbf{g}(y)\, d\sigma(y) ,$$

or equivalently,

$$\int_{\partial\Omega} \mathbf{N}(x,y)(-\frac{1}{2}I + \mathcal{K}^*_\Omega)\mathbf{g}(y)\, d\sigma(y) = \int_{\partial\Omega} \mathbf{\Gamma}(x-y)\mathbf{g}(y)\, d\sigma(y) , \quad x \in \Omega ,$$

for any $\mathbf{g} \in L^2_\psi(\partial\Omega)$. Consequently, it follows that, for any simply connected smooth domain D compactly contained in Ω and for any $\mathbf{g} \in L^2_\psi(\partial D)$, the following identity holds:

$$\int_{\partial D} (-\frac{1}{2}I + \mathcal{K}_\Omega)(\mathbf{N}_y)(x)\mathbf{g}(y)\, d\sigma(y) = \int_{\partial D} \mathbf{\Gamma}_y(x)\mathbf{g}(y)\, d\sigma(y) ,$$

for all $x \in \partial\Omega$. Therefore, the following lemma has been proved.

Lemma 3.3.11 *For $y \in \Omega$ and $x \in \partial\Omega$, let $\mathbf{\Gamma}_y(x) := \mathbf{\Gamma}(x-y)$ and $\mathbf{N}_y(x) := \mathbf{N}(x,y)$. Then*

$$\left(-\frac{1}{2}I + \mathcal{K}_\Omega \right)(\mathbf{N}_y)(x) = \mathbf{\Gamma}_y(x) \quad modulo \ \Psi . \tag{3.101}$$

We fix now some notation. Let

$$N_D\mathbf{f}(x) := \int_{\partial D} \mathbf{N}(x,y)\mathbf{f}(y)\, d\sigma(y) , \quad x \in \overline{\Omega} .$$

Theorem 3.3.12 *Let $\mathbf{u}$ be the solution to (3.88) and $\mathbf{U}$ the background solution, i.e., the solution to (3.83). Then the following holds:*

$$\mathbf{u}(x) = \mathbf{U}(x) - N_D\psi(x), \quad x \in \partial\Omega , \tag{3.102}$$

where ψ is defined by (3.95).

Proof. By substituting (3.93) into the equation (3.94), we obtain

$$\mathbf{H}(x) = -\mathcal{S}_\Omega(\mathbf{g})(x) + \mathcal{D}_\Omega\Big(\mathbf{H}|_{\partial\Omega} + (\mathcal{S}_D\psi)|_{\partial\Omega}\Big)(x) , \quad x \in \Omega .$$

By using (3.77), we see that

$$(\frac{1}{2}I - \mathcal{K}_\Omega)(\mathbf{H}|_{\partial\Omega}) = -(\mathcal{S}_\Omega\mathbf{g})|_{\partial\Omega} + (\frac{1}{2}I + \mathcal{K}_\Omega)((\mathcal{S}_D\psi)|_{\partial\Omega}) \quad \text{on } \partial\Omega . \quad (3.103)$$

Since $\mathbf{U}(x) = -\mathcal{S}_\Omega(\mathbf{g})(x) + \mathcal{D}_\Omega(\mathbf{U}|_{\partial\Omega})(x)$ for all $x \in \Omega$, we have

$$(\frac{1}{2}I - \mathcal{K}_\Omega)(\mathbf{U}|_{\partial\Omega}) = -(\mathcal{S}_\Omega\mathbf{g})|_{\partial\Omega} . \quad (3.104)$$

By Theorem 3.3.8 and (3.101), we have

$$(-\frac{1}{2}I + \mathcal{K}_\Omega)((N_D\psi)|_{\partial\Omega})(x) = (\mathcal{S}_D\psi)(x) , \quad x \in \partial\Omega , \quad (3.105)$$

since $\psi \in L^2_{\bar\Psi}(\partial D)$. We see from (3.103), (3.104), and (3.105) that

$$(\frac{1}{2}I - \mathcal{K}_\Omega)\Big(\mathbf{H}|_{\partial\Omega} - \mathbf{U}|_{\partial\Omega} + (\frac{1}{2}I + \mathcal{K}_\Omega)((N_D\psi)|_{\partial\Omega})\Big) = 0 \quad \text{on } \partial\Omega ,$$

and hence, by Corollary 3.3.7, we obtain that

$$\mathbf{H}|_{\partial\Omega} - \mathbf{U}|_{\partial\Omega} + (\frac{1}{2}I + \mathcal{K}_\Omega)((N_D\psi)|_{\partial\Omega}) \in \Psi .$$

Note that

$$(\frac{1}{2}I + \mathcal{K}_\Omega)((N_D\psi)|_{\partial\Omega}) = (N_D\psi)|_{\partial\Omega} + (\mathcal{S}_D\psi)|_{\partial\Omega} ,$$

which follows from (3.101). Thus, (3.93) gives

$$\mathbf{u}|_{\partial\Omega} = \mathbf{U}|_{\partial\Omega} - (N_D\psi)|_{\partial\Omega} \quad \text{modulo } \Psi . \quad (3.106)$$

Since all the functions in (3.106) belong to $L^2_{\bar\Psi}(\partial\Omega)$, we have (3.102). This completes the proof. □

3.4 Dynamic Elasticity

Consider the elastic wave equation $\partial_t^2\mathbf{U} - \mathcal{L}_{\lambda,\mu}\mathbf{U} = 0$. We obtain a time-harmonic solution $\mathbf{U}(x,t) = \Re e[e^{-i\omega t}\mathbf{u}(x)]$ if the space-dependent part $\mathbf{u}$ satisfies the equation, $(\mathcal{L}_{\lambda,\mu} + \omega^2)\mathbf{u} = 0$.

We begin this section by establishing the radiation condition for the elastic waves. This condition reduces to Sommerfeld radiation conditions for solutions of two Helmholtz equations. Then we give formulae for the fundamental solutions in the two- and three-dimensional cases. After that, the single- and double layer potentials are defined and the transmission is investigated. Due to the singular character of the kernels, the properties of these potentials are completely analogous to those associated with the static elasticity. The decomposition formula (3.3.10) is extended to the dynamic case. The method of derivation is parallel to that in the static case.

3.4.1 Radiation Condition

First, let us formulate the *radiation conditions* for the elastic waves when $\Im m\, \omega \geq 0$ and $\omega \neq 0$. Denote by

$$c_L = \sqrt{\lambda + 2\mu}, \quad c_T = \sqrt{\mu} \,.$$

Any solution $\mathbf{u}$ to $(\mathcal{L}_{\lambda,\mu} + \omega^2)\mathbf{u} = 0$ admits the decomposition, see [85, Theorem 2.5],

$$\mathbf{u} = \mathbf{u}^{(L)} + \mathbf{u}^{(T)} \,, \tag{3.107}$$

where $\mathbf{u}^{(L)}$ and $\mathbf{u}^{(T)}$ are given by

$$\mathbf{u}^{(L)} = (k_T^2 - k_L^2)^{-1}(\triangle + k_T^2)\mathbf{u} \,,$$
$$\mathbf{u}^{(T)} = (k_L^2 - k_T^2)^{-1}(\triangle + k_L^2)\mathbf{u} \,,$$

with $k_L = \omega/c_L$ and $k_T = \omega/c_T$. Then $\mathbf{u}^{(L)}$ and $\mathbf{u}^{(T)}$ satisfy the equations

$$\begin{cases} (\triangle + k_L^2)\mathbf{u}^{(L)} = 0 \,, & \nabla \times \mathbf{u}^{(L)} = 0 \,, \\ (\triangle + k_T^2)\mathbf{u}^{(T)} = 0 \,, & \nabla \cdot \mathbf{u}^{(T)} = 0 \,. \end{cases} \tag{3.108}$$

We impose on $\mathbf{u}^{(L)}$ and $\mathbf{u}^{(T)}$ the Sommerfeld radiation conditions for solutions of the Helmholtz equations by requiring that

$$\begin{cases} \partial_r \mathbf{u}^{(L)}(x) - ik_L \mathbf{u}^{(L)}(x) = o(r^{-(d-1)/2}) \\ \partial_r \mathbf{u}^{(T)}(x) - ik_T \mathbf{u}^{(T)}(x) = o(r^{-(d-1)/2}) \end{cases} \quad \text{as } r = |x| \to +\infty \,. \tag{3.109}$$

We say that $\mathbf{u}$ satisfies the radiation condition if it allows the decomposition (3.107) with $\mathbf{u}^{(L)}$ and $\mathbf{u}^{(T)}$ satisfying (3.108) and (3.109).

3.4.2 Fundamental Solution

We first consider the three-dimensional case. The Kupradze matrix $\Gamma^\omega = (\Gamma_{ij}^\omega)_{i,j=1}^3$ of the fundamental outgoing solution to the operator $\mathcal{L}_{\lambda,\mu} + \omega^2$ is given by

$$\Gamma_{ij}^\omega(x) = -\frac{\delta_{ij}}{4\pi\mu|x|} e^{\frac{i\omega|x|}{c_T}} + \frac{1}{4\pi\omega^2} \partial_i \partial_j \frac{e^{\frac{i\omega|x|}{c_L}} - e^{\frac{i\omega|x|}{c_T}}}{|x|} \,.$$

See [85, Chapter 2]. One can easily see that Γ_{ij}^ω allows the following expansion:

$$\Gamma_{ij}^\omega(x) = -\frac{1}{4\pi} \sum_{n=0}^{+\infty} \frac{i^n}{(n+2)n!} \left(\frac{n+1}{c_T^{n+2}} + \frac{1}{c_L^{n+2}} \right) \omega^n \delta_{ij} |x|^{n-1} \tag{3.110}$$

$$+ \frac{1}{4\pi} \sum_{n=0}^{+\infty} \frac{i^n(n-1)}{(n+2)n!} \left(\frac{1}{c_T^{n+2}} - \frac{1}{c_L^{n+2}} \right) \omega^n |x|^{n-3} x_i x_j \,.$$

If $\omega = 0$, then $\boldsymbol{\Gamma}^0$ is the Kelvin matrix of the fundamental solution to the Lamé system, given by (3.70) for $d = 3$.

In the two-dimensional case, the fundamental outgoing solution $\boldsymbol{\Gamma}^\omega$ is given by

$$
\begin{aligned}
\Gamma_{ij}^\omega(x) = &-\frac{i}{4\mu}\delta_{ij}H_0^{(1)}\left(\frac{\omega\sqrt{\rho}|x|}{c_p}\right) \\
&+\frac{i}{4\omega^2\rho}\partial_i\partial_j\left(H_0^{(1)}\left(\frac{\omega\sqrt{\rho}|x|}{c_s}\right) - H_0^{(1)}\left(\frac{\omega\sqrt{\rho}|x|}{c_p}\right)\right) ,
\end{aligned}
\tag{3.111}
$$

where $H_0^{(1)}$ is the Hankel function of the first kind and of order 0. For $\omega = 0$, again we set $\boldsymbol{\Gamma}^0$ to be the Kelvin matrix of the fundamental solution to the Lamé system.

3.4.3 Layer Potentials

The single- and double-layer potentials are defined by

$$
\mathcal{S}_\Omega^\omega\varphi(x) = \int_{\partial\Omega}\boldsymbol{\Gamma}^\omega(x-y)\varphi(y)d\sigma(y) ,
\tag{3.112}
$$

$$
\mathcal{D}_\Omega^\omega\varphi(x) = \int_{\partial\Omega}\frac{\partial}{\partial\nu_y}\boldsymbol{\Gamma}^\omega(x-y)\varphi(y)d\sigma(y) ,
\tag{3.113}
$$

for any $\varphi \in L^2(\partial\Omega)$. The following formulae give the jump relations obeyed by the double layer potential and by the conormal derivative of the single layer potential:

$$
\frac{\partial(\mathcal{S}_\Omega^\omega\varphi)}{\partial\nu}\bigg|_\pm(x) = \left(\pm\frac{1}{2}I + (\mathcal{K}_\Omega^\omega)^*\right)\varphi(x) , \quad \text{a.e. } x \in \partial\Omega ,
\tag{3.114}
$$

$$
(\mathcal{D}_\Omega^\omega\varphi)\big|_\pm(x) = \left(\mp\frac{1}{2}I + \mathcal{K}_\Omega^\omega\right)\varphi(x) , \quad \text{a.e. } x \in \partial\Omega ,
\tag{3.115}
$$

where $\mathcal{K}_\Omega^\omega$ is the operator defined by

$$
\mathcal{K}_\Omega^\omega(x) = \text{p.v.} \int_{\partial\Omega}\frac{\partial\boldsymbol{\Gamma}^\omega(x-y)}{\partial\nu_y}\varphi(y)d\sigma(y) ,
\tag{3.116}
$$

and $(\mathcal{K}_\Omega^\omega)^*$ is the L^2-adjoint of $\mathcal{K}_\Omega^{-\omega}$, that is,

$$
(\mathcal{K}_\Omega^\omega)^*(x) = \text{p.v.} \int_{\partial\Omega}\frac{\partial\boldsymbol{\Gamma}^\omega(x-y)}{\partial\nu_x}\varphi(y)d\sigma(y) .
$$

By a straightforward calculation one can see that the single- and double-layer potentials satisfy the radiation condition (3.109). We refer to [85] for the details.

3.4.4 Transmission Problem

Let $\tilde{\lambda}, \tilde{\mu}$ be another pair of Lamé parameters such that (3.84) and (3.85) hold. Let $\tilde{\mathcal{S}}_D^\omega$ denote the single layer potential defined by (3.112) with λ, μ replaced by $\tilde{\lambda}, \tilde{\mu}$.

We now have the following solvability result which can be viewed as a compact perturbation of the static case $\omega = 0$.

Theorem 3.4.1 *Suppose that $(\lambda - \tilde{\lambda})(\mu - \tilde{\mu}) \geq 0$ and $0 < \tilde{\lambda}, \tilde{\mu} < +\infty$. Suppose that ω^2 is not a Dirichlet eigenvalue for $-\mathcal{L}_{\lambda,\mu}$ on D. For any given $(\mathbf{F}, \mathbf{G}) \in W_1^2(\partial D) \times L^2(\partial D)$, there exists a unique pair $(\mathbf{f}, \mathbf{g}) \in L^2(\partial D) \times L^2(\partial D)$ such that*

$$\begin{cases} \tilde{\mathcal{S}}_D^\omega \mathbf{f}|_- - \mathcal{S}_D^\omega \mathbf{g}|_+ = \mathbf{F}, \\ \dfrac{\partial}{\partial \tilde{\nu}} \tilde{\mathcal{S}}_D^\omega \mathbf{f}|_- - \dfrac{\partial}{\partial \nu} \mathcal{S}_D^\omega \mathbf{g}|_+ = \mathbf{G}. \end{cases}$$

If $\omega = 0$ and $\mathbf{G} \in L_\psi^2(\partial D)$, then $\mathbf{g} \in L_\psi^2(\partial D)$. Moreover, if $\mathbf{F} \in \Psi$ and $\mathbf{G} = 0$, then $\mathbf{g} = 0$.

Consider now the following transmission problem:

$$\begin{cases} \mathcal{L}_{\lambda,\mu} \mathbf{u} + \omega^2 \mathbf{u} = 0 & \text{in } \Omega \setminus \overline{D}, \\ \mathcal{L}_{\tilde{\lambda},\tilde{\mu}} \mathbf{u} + \omega^2 \mathbf{u} = 0 & \text{in } D, \\ \dfrac{\partial \mathbf{u}}{\partial \nu} = \mathbf{g} & \text{on } \partial \Omega, \\ \mathbf{u}|_+ - \mathbf{u}|_- = 0 & \text{on } \partial D, \\ \dfrac{\partial \mathbf{u}}{\partial \nu}\Big|_+ - \dfrac{\partial \mathbf{u}}{\partial \tilde{\nu}}\Big|_- = 0 & \text{on } \partial D. \end{cases} \tag{3.117}$$

For this problem we have the following decomposition formula.

Theorem 3.4.2 (Decomposition Formula) *Suppose that ω^2 is not a Dirichlet eigenvalue for $-\mathcal{L}_{\lambda,\mu}$ on D. Let $\mathbf{u}$ be a solution to (3.117) and $\mathbf{f} := \mathbf{u}|_{\partial\Omega}$. Define*

$$\mathbf{H}(x) := \mathcal{D}_\Omega^\omega(\mathbf{f})(x) - \mathcal{S}_\Omega^\omega(\mathbf{g})(x), \quad x \in \mathbb{R}^d \setminus \partial\Omega. \tag{3.118}$$

Then $\mathbf{u}$ can be represented as

$$\mathbf{u}(x) = \begin{cases} \mathbf{H}(x) + \mathcal{S}_D^\omega \psi(x), & x \in \Omega \setminus \overline{D}, \\ \tilde{\mathcal{S}}_D^\omega \phi(x), & x \in D, \end{cases} \tag{3.119}$$

where the pair $(\phi, \psi) \in L^2(\partial D) \times L^2(\partial D)$ is the unique solution to

$$\begin{cases} \tilde{\mathcal{S}}_D^\omega \phi - \mathcal{S}_D^\omega \psi = \mathbf{H}|_{\partial D}, \\ \dfrac{\partial}{\partial \tilde{\nu}} \tilde{\mathcal{S}}_D^\omega \phi - \dfrac{\partial}{\partial \nu} \mathcal{S}_D^\omega \psi = \dfrac{\partial \mathbf{H}}{\partial \nu}\Big|_{\partial D}. \end{cases} \tag{3.120}$$

Moreover, we have

$$\mathbf{H}(x) + \mathcal{S}_D^\omega \psi(x) = 0, \quad x \in \mathbb{R}^d \setminus \overline{\Omega}. \tag{3.121}$$

Proof. We consider the following two phases transmission problem:

$$
\begin{cases}
\mathcal{L}_{\lambda,\mu}\mathbf{v} + \omega^2\mathbf{v} = 0 & \text{in } (\Omega \setminus \overline{D}) \bigcup (\mathbb{R}^d \setminus \overline{\Omega}) , \\
\mathcal{L}_{\tilde{\lambda},\tilde{\mu}}\mathbf{v} + \omega^2\mathbf{v} = 0 & \text{in } D , \\
\mathbf{v}\big|_{-} - \mathbf{v}\big|_{+} = \mathbf{f}, \quad \dfrac{\partial\mathbf{v}}{\partial\nu}\Big|_{-} - \dfrac{\partial\mathbf{v}}{\partial\nu}\Big|_{+} = \mathbf{g} & \text{on } \partial\Omega , \\
\mathbf{v}\big|_{-} - \mathbf{v}\big|_{+} = 0, \quad \dfrac{\partial\mathbf{v}}{\partial\tilde{\nu}}\Big|_{-} - \dfrac{\partial\mathbf{v}}{\partial\nu}\Big|_{+} = 0 & \text{on } \partial D ,
\end{cases}
\tag{3.122}
$$

with the radiation condition. This problem has a unique solution. See [85, Chapter 3]. It is easily checked that both $\mathbf{v}$ and $\tilde{\mathbf{v}}$ defined by

$$
\mathbf{v}(x) = \begin{cases} \mathbf{u}(x), & x \in \Omega , \\ 0, & x \in \mathbb{R}^d \setminus \overline{\Omega} , \end{cases} \quad \text{and} \quad \tilde{\mathbf{v}}(x) = \begin{cases} \mathbf{H}(x) + \mathcal{S}_D^\omega \psi(x) , & x \in \Omega \setminus \overline{D}, \\ \tilde{\mathcal{S}}_D^\omega \phi(x), & x \in D , \end{cases}
$$

are solutions to (3.122). Hence $\mathbf{v} = \tilde{\mathbf{v}}$. This completes the proof. □

3.5 Modified Stokes System

Consider the propagation of elastic waves in biological tissues. Let $\mathbf{u}$ be the displacement field, and (λ, μ) be the Lamé coefficients of the tissue. By (3.107), the elasticity system $(\mathcal{L}_{\lambda,\mu} + \omega^2)\mathbf{u} = 0$ can be split into two parts: $\mathbf{u} = \mathbf{u}^{(T)} + \mathbf{u}^{(L)}$; a null divergence solution $\mathbf{u}^{(T)}$ (shear waves) and a non-rotational solution $\mathbf{u}^{(L)}$ (compression waves) having respective propagation speeds of $c_T = \sqrt{\mu}$ and $c_L = \sqrt{\lambda + 2\mu}$. These two waves interact via mode conversation at boundaries and interfaces. The quasi-incompressibility of biological tissues leads to $\lambda \gg \mu$ and thus the compression waves $\mathbf{u}^{(L)}$ propagate much faster than the shear waves $\mathbf{u}^{(T)}$. To remove the compression modulus from consideration, we reduce in this case, as will be shown later, the elasticity system to a modified Stokes system.

In this section, we give a fundamental solution to the modified Stokes system, construct potentials associated with the modified Stokes system, investigate their mapping properties and jump relations, and use them to solve the transmission problem. We also prove a decomposition formula analogous to the ones derived in the preceding sections for the solution to the transmission problem. The theory of potentials associated with the modified Stokes system differs from the theory of potentials associated with linear elasticity only in the concrete analytical form of its potentials.

3.5.1 Fundamental Solution

For simplicity we treat only the three-dimensional case, leaving the derivations in two dimensions to the reader.

We consider the so-called modified Stokes system, *i.e.*, the problem of determining $\mathbf{v}$ and q in a domain Ω from the conditions:

$$\begin{cases} (\Delta + \kappa^2)\mathbf{v} - \nabla q = 0 \,, \\ \nabla \cdot \mathbf{v} = 0 \,, \\ \mathbf{v}|_{\partial\Omega} = \mathbf{g} \,. \end{cases} \qquad (3.123)$$

If $\kappa = 0$, then (3.123) becomes the standard Stokes system and we may regard (3.123) as a compact perturbation of that system.

Fundamental tensors $\mathbf{\Gamma}^\kappa = (\Gamma_{ij}^\kappa)_{i,j=1}^3$ and $\mathbf{F} = (F_i)_{i=1}^3$ to (3.123) in three dimensions are given by

$$\begin{cases} \Gamma_{ij}^\kappa(x) = -\dfrac{\delta_{ij}}{4\pi} \dfrac{e^{i\kappa|x|}}{|x|} - \dfrac{1}{4\pi\kappa^2} \partial_i \partial_j \dfrac{e^{i\kappa|x|} - 1}{|x|} \,, \\ F_i(x) = -\dfrac{1}{4\pi} \dfrac{x_i}{|x|^3} \,. \end{cases} \qquad (3.124)$$

In fact, since $e^{i\kappa|x|}/(4\pi|x|)$ is a fundamental solution to the Helmholtz operator $\Delta + \kappa^2$ and

$$\partial_i \partial_j \frac{e^{i\kappa|x|} - 1}{|x|} = \sum_{k=1}^\infty \frac{(i\kappa)^{k+1}}{(k+1)!} \left[k(k-2)|x|^{k-4} x_i x_j + k\delta_{ij}|x|^{k-2} \right], \qquad (3.125)$$

we have

$$\begin{cases} (\Delta + \kappa^2)\Gamma_{ij}^\kappa - \partial_j F_i = \delta_{ij}\delta_0 \\ \partial_i \Gamma_{ij}^\kappa = 0 \end{cases} \quad \text{in } \mathbb{R}^3$$

in the sense of distributions. Note that we used the Einstein convention for the summation notation omitting the summation sign for the indices appearing twice. We will continue using this convention throughout this book. Moreover, we have from (3.125) that

$$\Gamma_{ij}^\kappa(x) = \Gamma_{ij}^0(x) + O(\kappa) \qquad (3.126)$$

uniformly in x as long as $|x|$ is bounded, where

$$\Gamma_{ij}^0(x) = -\frac{1}{8\pi} \left(\frac{\delta_{ij}}{|x|} + \frac{x_i x_j}{|x|^3} \right) \,. \qquad (3.127)$$

It is known (see for example [90]) that $\mathbf{\Gamma}^0 = (\Gamma_{ij}^0)_{i,j=1}^3$ and $\mathbf{F}$ are the fundamental tensors for the standard Stokes system. We refer to Ladyzhenskaya [90, Chapter 3] for a complete treatment of the theory of potentials associated with the Stokes system.

3.5.2 Layer Potentials

Introduce the single- and double-layer potentials on ∂D. For $i = 1, 2, 3$, $\varphi = (\varphi_1, \varphi_2, \varphi_3) \in L^2(\partial D)$, and for $x \in \mathbb{R}^3 \setminus \partial D$, let

$$\begin{cases} \mathcal{S}_D^\kappa[\varphi]_i(x) := \displaystyle\int_{\partial D} \Gamma_{ij}^\kappa(x-y)\varphi_j(y)\, d\sigma(y)\,, \\[2mm] \mathcal{Q}_D[\varphi](x) := \displaystyle\int_{\partial D} F_j(x-y)\varphi_j(y)\, d\sigma(y)\,, \end{cases}$$

and

$$\begin{cases} \mathcal{D}_D^\kappa[\varphi]_i(x) := \displaystyle\int_{\partial D} \left(\frac{\partial \Gamma_{ij}^\kappa}{\partial \mathbf{N}(y)}(x-y) + F_i(x-y)N_j(y)\right)\varphi_j(y)\, d\sigma(y)\,, \\[3mm] \mathcal{V}_D[\varphi](x) := -2\displaystyle\int_{\partial D} \frac{\partial}{\partial x_l} F_j(x-y)\varphi_j(y)N_l(y)\, d\sigma(y)\,. \end{cases}$$

By abuse of notation, let

$$\frac{\partial \mathbf{u}}{\partial \mathbf{N}} = (\nabla \mathbf{u} + \nabla \mathbf{u}^T)\mathbf{N}\,.$$

Note that

$$\frac{\partial \Gamma_{ij}^\kappa}{\partial \mathbf{N}(y)}(x-y) = \left(\frac{\partial \Gamma_{ij}^\kappa(x-y)}{\partial y_l} + \frac{\partial \Gamma_{il}^\kappa(x-y)}{\partial y_j}\right)N_l(y)\,.$$

Then $(\mathcal{S}_D^\kappa[\varphi], \mathcal{Q}_D[\varphi])$ and $(\mathcal{D}_D^\kappa[\varphi], \mathcal{V}_D[\varphi])$ satisfy (3.123).

We define the conormal derivative $\partial/\partial n$ by

$$\frac{\partial \mathbf{v}}{\partial n}\bigg|_{\pm} = \frac{\partial \mathbf{v}}{\partial \mathbf{N}}\bigg|_{\pm} - q\big|_{\pm}\,\mathbf{N} \quad \text{on } \partial D$$

for a pair $(\mathbf{v}, q)$. Then, for any pairs $(\mathbf{u}, p)$ and $(\mathbf{v}, q)$ satisfying $\nabla \cdot \mathbf{u} = 0$ and $\nabla \cdot \mathbf{v} = 0$, the following Green formulae hold (see [90]):

$$\int_{\partial D} \mathbf{u} \cdot \frac{\partial \mathbf{v}}{\partial n}\, d\sigma = \int_D \frac{1}{2}\sum_{i,j=1}^{3}\left(\frac{\partial u_i}{\partial x_j} + \frac{\partial u_j}{\partial x_i}\right)\left(\frac{\partial v_i}{\partial x_j} + \frac{\partial v_j}{\partial x_i}\right) + \mathbf{u}\cdot(\triangle\mathbf{v} - \nabla q)\, dx,$$

$$\int_{\partial D}\left(\mathbf{u}\cdot\frac{\partial \mathbf{v}}{\partial n} - \mathbf{v}\cdot\frac{\partial \mathbf{u}}{\partial n}\right) d\sigma = \int_D \mathbf{u}\cdot(\triangle\mathbf{v} - \nabla q) - \mathbf{v}\cdot(\triangle\mathbf{u} - \nabla p)\, dx\,.$$

We also obtain a representation formula for a solution $(\mathbf{v}, q)$ to (3.124):

$$\begin{cases} \mathbf{v}(x) = -\mathcal{S}_D^\kappa\left[\dfrac{\partial \mathbf{v}}{\partial n}\big|_{-}\right](x) + \mathcal{D}_D^\kappa[\mathbf{v}](x)\,, \\[3mm] q(x) = -\mathcal{Q}_D\left[\dfrac{\partial \mathbf{v}}{\partial n}\big|_{-}\right](x) + \mathcal{V}_D[\mathbf{v}](x)\,, \end{cases} \quad x \in D\,.$$

For $\varphi \in L^2(\partial D)$, the following trace relations for $\mathcal{D}_D^\kappa$ and the conormal derivative of $\mathcal{S}_D^\kappa$ hold:

$$\mathcal{D}_D^\kappa[\varphi]\big|_{\pm} = (\mp\frac{1}{2}I + \mathcal{K}_D^\kappa)[\varphi] \quad \text{a.e. on } \partial D\,, \tag{3.128}$$

$$\frac{\partial}{\partial n}\mathcal{S}_D^\kappa[\varphi]\bigg|_{\pm} = (\pm\frac{1}{2}I + (\mathcal{K}_D^\kappa)^*)[\varphi] \quad \text{a.e. on } \partial D\,, \tag{3.129}$$

where $\mathcal{K}_D^\kappa$ is defined by

$$
\begin{aligned}
\mathcal{K}_D^\kappa[\varphi]_i(x) := \ &\mathrm{p.v.} \int_{\partial D} \frac{\partial \Gamma_{ij}^\kappa}{\partial \mathbf{N}(y)}(x-y)\varphi_j(y)\,d\sigma(y) \\
&+ \ \mathrm{p.v.} \int_{\partial D} F_i(x-y)\varphi_j(y)N_j(y)\,d\sigma(y) ,
\end{aligned}
\tag{3.130}
$$

for almost all $x \in \partial D$, and $(\mathcal{K}_D^\kappa)^*$ is the adjoint operator of $\mathcal{K}_D^{-\kappa}$ on $L^2(\partial D)$, that is,

$$
\begin{aligned}
(\mathcal{K}_D^\kappa)^*[\varphi]_i(x) := \ &\mathrm{p.v.} \int_{\partial D} \frac{\partial \Gamma_{ij}^\kappa}{\partial \mathbf{N}(x)}(x-y)\varphi_j(y)\,d\sigma(y) \\
&- \ \mathrm{p.v.} \int_{\partial D} F_i(x-y)\varphi_j(y)N_j(x)\,d\sigma(y) .
\end{aligned}
$$

In fact, formulae (3.128) and (3.129) were proved in [90] when $\kappa = 0$. Since $\mathcal{D}_D^\kappa - \mathcal{D}_D^0$ and $\mathcal{S}_D^\kappa - \mathcal{S}_D^0$ are smoothing operators according to (3.126), we obtain (3.128) and (3.129) when $\kappa \neq 0$. It would be of use to the reader to note that by putting together the two integrals in (3.130), we have

$$
\mathcal{K}_D^0[\varphi]_i(x) := -\frac{3}{4\pi} \int_{\partial D} \frac{\langle x-y, \mathbf{N}(y)\rangle (x_i - y_i)(x_j - y_j)}{|x-y|^5}\varphi_j(y)d\sigma(y) . \tag{3.131}
$$

If ∂D is C^2 as we assume it to be, then

$$
|\langle x-y, \mathbf{N}(y)\rangle| \leq C|x-y|^2 , \tag{3.132}
$$

and hence $\mathcal{K}_D^0$ is a compact operator on $L^2(\partial D)$.

Formulae (3.128) and (3.129) show, in particular, that the double and single layer potentials obey the following jump relations on ∂D:

$$
\mathcal{D}_D^\kappa[\varphi]|_+ - \mathcal{D}_D^\kappa[\varphi]|_- = -\varphi \quad \text{a.e. on } \partial D , \tag{3.133}
$$

$$
\frac{\partial}{\partial n}\mathcal{S}_D^\kappa[\varphi]\Big|_+ - \frac{\partial}{\partial n}\mathcal{S}_D^\kappa[\varphi]\Big|_- = \varphi \quad \text{a.e. on } \partial D . \tag{3.134}
$$

On the other hand, the conormal derivative of the double layer potentials does not have a jump. In fact, if $\varphi \in W_1^2(\partial D)$ then

$$
\begin{aligned}
\frac{\partial}{\partial n}(\mathcal{D}_D^\kappa[\varphi])_i\Big|_+ (x) &= \frac{\partial}{\partial n}(\mathcal{D}_D^\kappa[\varphi])_i\Big|_- (x) \\
&= \mathrm{p.v.} \int_{\partial D} \frac{\partial^2 \Gamma_{ij}^\kappa}{\partial \mathbf{N}(x)\partial \mathbf{N}(y)}(x-y)\varphi_j(y)\,d\sigma(y)
\end{aligned}
\tag{3.135}
$$

a.e. on ∂D.

Lemma 3.5.1 (Mapping Properties) *Let $L_0^2(\partial D) := \{\mathbf{g} \in L^2(\partial D) : \int_{\partial D} \mathbf{g} \cdot \mathbf{N} = 0\}$, and define $(W_1^2)_0(\partial D)$ likewise. Let $L := Ker\left(\frac{1}{2}I + \mathcal{K}_D^0\right)^{\perp}$ in $L^2(\partial D)$. Then the following holds:*

(i) $\mathcal{S}_D^0 : L_0^2(\partial D) \to (W_1^2)_0(\partial D)$ is invertible.
(ii) $\frac{1}{2}I + \mathcal{K}_D^0 : L \to L_0^2(\partial D)$ is invertible and so is $\frac{1}{2}I + (\mathcal{K}_D^0)^* : L_0^2(\partial D) \to L$.
(iii) $\lambda I + \mathcal{K}_D^0$ and $\lambda I + (\mathcal{K}_D^0)^*$ are invertible on $L^2(\partial D)$ for $|\lambda| > 1/2$.

Proof. The assertion (ii) was proved in [90]. We also recall from [90] that

$$\mathrm{Ker}\mathcal{S}_D^0 = \mathrm{Ker}\left(\frac{1}{2}I + (\mathcal{K}_D^0)^*\right) = \langle \mathbf{N} \rangle , \qquad (3.136)$$

where $\mathbf{N}$ is the outward normal to ∂D.

To prove (i), let $\mathbf{g} \in (W_1^2)_0(\partial D)$ and $\mathbf{v}$ be the solution to the exterior problem for the Stokes system, *i.e.*,

$$\begin{cases} \Delta\mathbf{v} - \nabla q = 0 & \text{in } \mathbb{R}^3 \setminus \overline{D} , \\ \nabla \cdot \mathbf{v} = 0 & \text{in } \mathbb{R}^3 \setminus \overline{D} , \\ \mathbf{v} = \mathbf{g} & \text{on } \partial D , \\ \mathbf{v}(x) = O(|x|^{-2}) & \text{as } |x| \to \infty . \end{cases} \qquad (3.137)$$

Let $\phi \in L^2(\partial D)$ satisfy $(\frac{1}{2}I + \mathcal{K}_D^0)[\phi] = 0$ on ∂D. Then, because of (3.132), we have $\mathcal{K}_D^0\phi \in W_1^2(\partial D)$, and hence $\phi \in W_1^2(\partial D)$. Moreover, by (3.128), we have $\mathcal{D}_D^0[\phi] = 0$ in D, and the corresponding pressure $q = c$ in D for some constant c. It thus follows from (3.136) and (3.135) that

$$\left.\frac{\partial\mathcal{D}_D^0[\phi]}{\partial n}\right|_+ = \left.\frac{\partial\mathcal{D}_D^0[\phi]}{\partial n}\right|_- = \left.\frac{\partial\mathcal{D}_D^0[\phi]}{\partial \mathbf{N}}\right|_- - q|_-\mathbf{N} = -c\mathbf{N} .$$

Applying Green's formula, we have

$$\int_{\partial D} \frac{\partial\mathbf{v}}{\partial n} \cdot \phi = -\int_{\partial D} \frac{\partial\mathbf{v}}{\partial n} \cdot \left(-\frac{1}{2}I + \mathcal{K}_D^0\right)\phi = -\int_{\partial D} \mathbf{v} \cdot \left.\frac{\partial\mathcal{D}_D^0[\phi]}{\partial n}\right|_+ = 0 .$$

Thus

$$\frac{\partial\mathbf{v}}{\partial n} \in L .$$

Let

$$\psi := \left(\frac{1}{2}I + (\mathcal{K}_D^0)^*\right)^{-1}\left[\frac{\partial\mathbf{v}}{\partial n}\right] \quad \text{on } \partial D .$$

Then, by (3.129), we get

$$\left.\frac{\partial(\mathcal{S}_D^0[\psi])}{\partial n}\right|_+ = \left.\frac{\partial\mathbf{v}}{\partial n}\right|_+ ,$$

and hence $\mathcal{S}_D^0[\psi] = \mathbf{v}$ in $\mathbb{R}^3 \setminus D$. In particular, $\mathcal{S}_D^0[\psi] = \mathbf{g}$ and hence $\mathcal{S}_D^0 :$ $L_0^2(\partial D) \to (W_1^2)_0(\partial D)$ is onto. Therefore we obtain (i).

To prove (iii), suppose that $\left(\lambda I + (\mathcal{K}_D^0)^*\right)[\phi] = 0$ on ∂D. By Green's formula, we have

$$\frac{1}{2} \int_D \sum_{i,k=1}^3 \left(\frac{\partial \mathcal{S}_D^0[\phi]_i}{\partial x_k} + \frac{\partial \mathcal{S}_D^0[\phi]_k}{\partial x_i}\right)^2 dx = \int_{\partial D} \left(-\frac{1}{2}I + (\mathcal{K}_D^0)^*\right)[\phi] \cdot \mathcal{S}_D^0[\phi] d\sigma$$

$$= \frac{\lambda + \frac{1}{2}}{\lambda - \frac{1}{2}} \int_{\partial D} \left(\frac{1}{2}I + (\mathcal{K}_D^0)^*\right)[\phi] \cdot \mathcal{S}_D^0[\phi] d\sigma$$

$$= -\frac{1}{2}\frac{\lambda + \frac{1}{2}}{\lambda - \frac{1}{2}} \int_{\mathbb{R}^3 \setminus \overline{D}} \sum_{i,k=1}^3 \left(\frac{\partial \mathcal{S}_D^0[\phi]_i}{\partial x_k} + \frac{\partial \mathcal{S}_D^0[\phi]_k}{\partial x_i}\right)^2 dx \ .$$

Since $(\lambda + (1/2))/(\lambda - (1/2)) > 0$, we have

$$\frac{\partial \mathcal{S}_D^0[\phi]_i}{\partial x_k} + \frac{\partial \mathcal{S}_D^0[\phi]_k}{\partial x_i} = 0 \quad \text{in } \mathbb{R}^3 \setminus \partial D, \quad i,j = 1,2,3 \ , \tag{3.138}$$

which implies that $\mathcal{S}_D^0[\phi] = C$ in $\mathbb{R}^3 \setminus \overline{D}$ for some constant C. On the other hand, $\mathcal{S}_D^0[\phi]$ vanishes at infinity, and hence it vanishes in $\mathbb{R}^3$. Therefore, we have

$$\phi = \frac{1}{\lambda - \frac{1}{2}} \left(\left(\lambda I + (\mathcal{K}_D^0)^*\right)\phi - \left(\frac{1}{2}I + (\mathcal{K}_D^0)^*\right)\phi\right) = 0 \ .$$

Thus $\left(\lambda I + (\mathcal{K}_D^0)^*\right)$ is injective on $L^2(\partial D)$. Since $(\mathcal{K}_D^0)^*$ is compact on $L^2(\partial D)$ by (3.132), we have (iii) by the Fredholm alternative. This completes the proof.
□

3.5.3 Transmission Problem

Suppose that $\int_{\partial\Omega} \mathbf{g} \cdot \mathbf{N} = 0$. Let μ and $\tilde{\mu}$ be two positive constants. Consider the transmission problem

$$\begin{cases} (\Delta + \kappa^2)\mathbf{u} - \nabla q = 0 & \text{in } \Omega \setminus \overline{D} \ , \\ (\Delta + \tilde{\kappa}^2)\mathbf{u} - \nabla q = 0 & \text{in } D \ , \\ \mathbf{u}\big|_+ - \mathbf{u}\big|_- = 0 & \text{on } \partial D \ , \\ \mu\dfrac{\partial \mathbf{u}}{\partial n}\bigg|_+ - \tilde{\mu}\dfrac{\partial \mathbf{u}}{\partial n}\bigg|_- = 0 & \text{on } \partial D \ , \\ \nabla \cdot \mathbf{u} = 0 & \text{in } \Omega \ , \\ \mathbf{u} = \mathbf{g} & \text{on } \partial\Omega \ , \\ \displaystyle\int_\Omega q = 0 \ . \end{cases} \tag{3.139}$$

We look for the solution to (3.139) in the form of

$$
\mathbf{u} = \begin{cases} \mathcal{S}_D^{\tilde{\kappa}}[\phi] & \text{in } D, \\ \mathcal{S}_D^{\kappa}[\psi] + \mathcal{D}_\Omega^{\kappa}[\theta] & \text{in } \Omega \setminus \overline{D} \end{cases} \tag{3.140}
$$

for some triplet $(\phi, \psi, \theta) \in L^2(\partial D) \times L^2(\partial D) \times L^2(\partial\Omega)$. Then (ϕ, ψ, θ) should satisfy the following system of integral equations:

$$
\begin{cases} \mathcal{S}_D^{\tilde{\kappa}}[\phi] - \mathcal{S}_D^{\kappa}[\psi] - \mathcal{D}_\Omega^{\kappa}[\theta] = 0 & \text{on } \partial D, \\ \tilde{\mu}(-\dfrac{1}{2}I + (\mathcal{K}_D^{\tilde{\kappa}})^*)[\phi] - \mu(\dfrac{1}{2}I + (\mathcal{K}_D^{\kappa})^*)[\psi] - \dfrac{\partial}{\partial n}\mathcal{D}_\Omega^{\kappa}[\theta] = 0 & \text{on } \partial D, \\ \mathcal{S}_D^{\kappa}[\psi] + (\dfrac{1}{2}I + \mathcal{K}_\Omega^{\kappa})[\theta] = \mathbf{g} & \text{on } \partial\Omega, \end{cases}
$$

or

$$
\begin{pmatrix} \mathcal{S}_D^{\tilde{\kappa}} & -\mathcal{S}_D^{\kappa} & -\mathcal{D}_\Omega^{\kappa} \\ \tilde{\mu}(-\frac{1}{2}I + (\mathcal{K}_D^{\tilde{\kappa}})^*) & -\mu(\frac{1}{2}I + (\mathcal{K}_D^{\kappa})^*) & -\frac{\partial}{\partial n}\mathcal{D}_\Omega^{\kappa} \\ 0 & \mathcal{S}_D^{\kappa} & \frac{1}{2}I + \mathcal{K}_\Omega^{\kappa} \end{pmatrix} \begin{pmatrix} \phi \\ \psi \\ \theta \end{pmatrix} = \begin{pmatrix} 0 \\ 0 \\ \mathbf{g} \end{pmatrix}. \tag{3.141}
$$

Denote the operator in (3.141) by A_κ. Then A_κ maps $L^2(\partial D) \times L^2(\partial D) \times L^2(\partial\Omega)$ into $(W_1^2)_0(\partial D) \times L^2(\partial D) \times L_0^2(\partial\Omega)$.

We now investigate the solvability of the equation (3.141). Because of (3.126), A_κ is a compact perturbation of A_0, which is again a compact perturbation of

$$
\begin{pmatrix} \mathcal{S}_D^0 & -\mathcal{S}_D^0 & 0 \\ \tilde{\mu}(-\frac{1}{2}I + (\mathcal{K}_D^0)^*) & -\mu(\frac{1}{2}I + (\mathcal{K}_D^0)^*) & 0 \\ 0 & 0 & \frac{1}{2}I + \mathcal{K}_\Omega^0 \end{pmatrix}. \tag{3.142}
$$

Define $S := \{(\phi, \psi) \in L^2(\partial D) \times L^2(\partial D) : \phi - \psi \in L_0^2(\partial D)\}$. Denote Ker $\left(\frac{1}{2}I + \mathcal{K}_\Omega^{\kappa}\right)^{\perp}$ by L_κ. Then the following holds.

Lemma 3.5.2 *The operator $\mathbf{A}_0 : S \times L_0 \to (W_1^2)_0(\partial D) \times L^2(\partial D) \times L_0^2(\partial\Omega)$ is invertible. So is $A_\kappa : S \times L_\kappa$ into $(W_1^2)_0(\partial D) \times L^2(\partial D) \times L_0^2(\partial\Omega)$, provided that κ^2 is not a Dirichlet eigenvalue of the Stokes system on either D or Ω.*

Proof. Using Lemma 3.5.1, one can easily show that the operator in (3.142) is invertible. Since $\mathbf{A}_0$ is its compact perturbation, it suffices to show that $\mathbf{A}_0$ is injective according to the Fredholm alternative.

Suppose that there exists $(\phi_0, \psi_0, \theta_0) \in S \times L_0$ such that

$$
\mathbf{A}_0 \begin{bmatrix} \phi_0 \\ \psi_0 \\ \theta_0 \end{bmatrix} = 0.
$$

Then the function $\mathbf{v}$ defined by

$$\mathbf{v}(x) := \begin{cases} \mathcal{S}_D^0[\phi_0](x), & x \in D, \\ \mathcal{S}_D^0[\psi_0](x) + \mathcal{D}_\Omega^0[\theta_0](x), & x \in \Omega \setminus \overline{D}, \end{cases}$$

is a solution to (3.139) with $\kappa = \widetilde{\kappa} = 0$ and $\mathbf{g} = 0$. Since the solution to (3.139) with $\kappa = \widetilde{\kappa} = 0$ is unique, we have

$$\mathcal{S}_D^0[\phi_0] = 0 \quad \text{in } D, \tag{3.143}$$

$$\mathcal{S}_D^0[\psi_0] + \mathcal{D}_\Omega^0[\theta_0] = 0 \quad \text{in } \Omega \setminus \overline{D}. \tag{3.144}$$

Then (3.144) shows that $\mathcal{S}_D^0[\psi_0]$ can be extended to Ω as a solution to (3.123). Hence by (3.134) we obtain $\psi_0 = c\mathbf{N}$ for some constant c, and $\mathcal{D}_\Omega^0[\theta_0] = 0$ in Ω. By (3.128) and part (ii) in Lemma 3.5.1, we have $\theta_0 = 0$. On the other hand,

$$\phi_0 = \left. \frac{\partial \mathcal{S}_D^0[\phi_0]}{\partial n} \right|_+ - \left. \frac{\partial \mathcal{S}_D^0[\phi_0]}{\partial n} \right|_- = \left. \frac{\partial \mathcal{S}_D^0[\phi_0]}{\partial n} \right|_+ - \frac{\mu}{\widetilde{\mu}} \left. \frac{\partial \mathcal{S}_D^0[\psi_0]}{\partial n} \right|_+ = 0,$$

and thus $\psi_0 = 0$. Therefore, $\mathbf{A}_0$ is invertible.

Since the operator in (3.141) is a compact perturbation of $\mathbf{A}_0$, we can show that it is invertible in exactly the same manner under the assumption that κ^2 is not a Dirichlet eigenvalue of the Stokes system in either D or Ω. This completes the proof. □

Thus we obtain the following theorem.

Theorem 3.5.3 *Let $(\phi, \psi, \theta) \in S \times L_\kappa$ be the unique solution to (3.141). Then the solution $\mathbf{u}$ to (3.139) is represented by (3.140).*

Consider the following boundary-value problem for the modified Stokes system in the absence of the elastic anomaly:

$$\begin{cases} (\Delta + \kappa^2)\mathbf{v} + \nabla q = 0 & \text{in } \Omega, \\ \nabla \cdot \mathbf{v} = 0 & \text{in } \Omega, \\ \mathbf{v} = \mathbf{g} & \text{on } \partial\Omega, \\ \displaystyle\int_\Omega q = 0, \end{cases} \tag{3.145}$$

under the compatibility condition $\int_{\partial\Omega} \mathbf{g} \cdot \mathbf{N} = 0$.

Let

$$\theta_0 = (\frac{1}{2}I + \mathcal{K}_\Omega^\kappa)^{-1}[\mathbf{g}] \quad \text{on } \partial\Omega.$$

Then the solution $\mathbf{U}$ to (3.145) is given by

$$\mathbf{U}(x) = \mathcal{D}_\Omega^\kappa[\theta_0](x) = \mathcal{D}_\Omega^\kappa(\frac{1}{2}I + \mathcal{K}_\Omega^\kappa)^{-1}[\mathbf{g}](x), \quad x \in \Omega.$$

By (3.140), we have

$$\mathcal{D}_\Omega^\kappa(\frac{1}{2}I + \mathcal{K}_\Omega^\kappa)^{-1}[\mathbf{g} - \mathcal{S}_D^\kappa[\psi]|_{\partial\Omega}] = \mathcal{D}_\Omega^\kappa(\frac{1}{2}I + \mathcal{K}_\Omega^\kappa)^{-1}[\mathcal{D}_\Omega^\kappa[\theta]|_-]$$
$$= \mathcal{D}_\Omega^\kappa[\theta],$$

and hence we obtain

$$\mathbf{u}(x) = \mathbf{U}(x) + \mathcal{S}_D^\kappa[\psi](x) - \mathcal{D}_\Omega^\kappa(\frac{1}{2} + \mathcal{K}_\Omega^\kappa)^{-1}[\mathcal{S}_D^\kappa[\psi]|_{\partial\Omega}](x), \quad x \in \Omega\setminus\overline{D}. \quad (3.146)$$

Let $\mathbf{\Gamma}^\kappa = (G_{ij}^\kappa)_{i,j=1}^3$ be the the Dirichlet Green function for the operator in (3.123), i.e., for $y \in \Omega$,

$$\begin{cases} (\Delta_x + \kappa^2)G_{ij}^\kappa(x,y) - \dfrac{\partial F_i(x-y)}{\partial x_j} = \delta_{ij}\delta_y(x) \quad \text{in } \Omega, \\[2mm] \displaystyle\sum_{j=1}^3 \dfrac{\partial}{\partial x_j}G_{ij}^\kappa(x,y) = 0 \quad \text{in } \Omega, \\[2mm] G_{ij}^\kappa(x,y) = 0 \quad \text{on } \partial\Omega. \end{cases}$$

Define for $\mathbf{f} \in L_0^2(\partial D)$

$$\mathcal{G}_D^\kappa[\mathbf{f}](x) := \int_{\partial D} \mathbf{\Gamma}^\kappa(x,y)\mathbf{f}(y)\,d\sigma, \quad x \in \Omega.$$

Then the following identity holds:

$$\mathcal{G}_D^\kappa[\mathbf{f}](x) = \mathcal{S}_D^\kappa[\mathbf{f}](x) - \mathcal{D}_\Omega^\kappa(\frac{1}{2} + \mathcal{K}_\Omega^\kappa)^{-1}\mathcal{S}_D^\kappa[\mathbf{f}](x), \quad x \in \Omega.$$

In fact, by the definition of the Green function, we have

$$\mathbf{\Gamma}^\kappa(x,y) = \mathbf{\Gamma}^\kappa(x,y) - \mathcal{D}_\Omega^\kappa(\frac{1}{2} + \mathcal{K}_\Omega^\kappa)^{-1}[\mathbf{\Gamma}^\kappa(\,\cdot\,,y)](x), \quad x \in \Omega.$$

From (3.146), we obtain the following theorem.

Theorem 3.5.4 *Let $(\phi, \psi, \theta) \in S \times L_\kappa$ be the unique solution to (3.141). Then*

$$\mathbf{u}(x) = \mathbf{U}(x) + \mathcal{G}_D^\kappa[\psi](x), \quad x \in \Omega\setminus\overline{D}. \quad (3.147)$$

Bibliography and Discussion

The decomposition formula in Theorem 3.1.13 was proved in [75, 76, 78]. It seems to inherit geometric properties of the anomaly. Based on Theorem 3.1.13, Kang and Seo proved global uniqueness results for the inverse conductivity problem with one measurement when the conductivity anomaly is a disk or a ball in three-dimensional space [75, 77]. Theorem 3.3.8 is due to Escauriaza and Seo [53]. Most of the results on modified Stokes system are from [8]. The book by Nédélec [104] is an excellent reference on integral equations method. A complete treatment of the Helmholtz equation as well as the full time-harmonic Maxwell equations is provided there.

Part II

General Reconstruction Algorithms

4

Tomographic Imaging with Non-Diffracting Sources

Image reconstruction is an important topic of tomographic imaging because spatial information is encoded into the measured data during the data acquisition step. Depending on how spatial information is encoded into the measured data, the image reconstruction technique can vary considerably. In this chapter we deal with the mathematical basis of tomography with non-diffracting sources. We outline two fundamental image reconstruction problems for detailed discussion: (i) reconstruction from Fourier transform samples, and (ii) reconstruction from Radon transform samples. Many practical MRI data acquisition schemes lend themselves naturally to one of these two reconstruction problems while computed tomography (CT) produces data exclusively as a series of projections.

This chapter is organized as follows. First, some general issues in image reconstruction are discussed. Then the algorithms of Fourier reconstruction are described. Finally, image reconstruction from Radon transform data is discussed, starting with a description of the inverse Radon transform, which is followed by an exposition of the practical algorithms.

4.1 Imaging Equations of CT and MRI

4.1.1 Imaging Equation of CT

In CT, one probes an object with non-diffracting radiation, *e.g.*, X-rays for the human body. If I_0 is the intensity of the source, $a(x)$ the linear attenuation coefficient of the object at point x, L the ray along which the radiation propagates, and I the intensity past the object, then

$$I = I_0 e^{-\int_L a(x)\,dx} . \tag{4.1}$$

In the simplest case the ray L may be thought of as a straight line. Modeling L as a strip or cone, possibly with a weight factor to account for detector inhomogeneities, may be more appropriate. Equation (4.1) neglects the dependence of a with the energy (beam hardening effect) and other nonlinear phenomena (*e.g.*, partial volume effect). The mathematical problem in CT is to determine a from measurements of I for a large set of rays L. If L is simply the straight line connecting the source x_0 with the detector x_1, equation (4.1) gives rise to

$$\ln(\frac{I}{I_0}) = -\int_{x_0}^{x_1} a(x)\,dx\ .\tag{4.2}$$

The task is to compute a in a domain $\Omega \subset \mathbb{R}^2$ from the values of equation (4.2) where x_0 and x_1 run through certain subsets of $\partial\Omega$. Equation (4.2) is simply a reparametrization of the Radon transform R.

4.1.2 Imaging Equation of MRI

The physical phenomenon exploited in MRI is the precession of the spin of a proton in a magnetic field of strength H about the direction of that field. The frequency of this precession is the Larmor frequency γH where γ is the gyromagnetic ratio. By making the magnetic field H space-dependent in a controlled way, the local magnetization $M_0(x)$ (together with the relaxation times $T_1(x)$ and $T_2(x)$) can be imaged. The magnetization $M(x,t)$ caused by a magnetic field $H(x,t)$ satisfies the Bloch equation

$$\frac{\partial M}{\partial t} = \gamma M \times H - \frac{1}{T_2}(M_1 \mathbf{e}_1 + M_2 \mathbf{e}_2) - \frac{1}{T_1}(M_3 - M_0)\mathbf{e}_3\ .\tag{4.3}$$

Here, M_i is the i–th components of M and $\mathbf{e}_i$ is the i–th unit vector for $i = 1, 2, 3$. The significance of T_1, T_2, M_0 becomes apparent if we solve (4.3) for the static field $H = H_0 \mathbf{e}_3$ with initial values $M(x, 0) = M^0(x)$. Setting $\omega_0 = \gamma H_0$ leads to

$$M_1(x, t) = e^{-t/T_2}(M_1^0 \cos \omega_0 t + M_2^0 \sin \omega_0 t)\ ,$$
$$M_2(x, t) = e^{-t/T_2}(-M_1^0 \sin \omega_0 t + M_2^0 \cos \omega_0 t)\ ,$$
$$M_3(x, t) = e^{-t/T_1} M_3^0 + (1 - e^{-t/T_1})M_0\ .$$

Thus the magnetization rotates in the (x_1, x_2) plane with Larmor frequency ω_0 and returns to the equilibrium position $(0, 0, M_0)$ with speed controlled by T_2 in the (x_1, x_2) plane and T_1 in the x_3-direction.

In an MRI scanner, one generates a field

$$H(x, t) = (H_0 + G(t) \cdot x)\mathbf{e}_3 + H_1(t)(\cos(\omega_0 t)\mathbf{e}_1 + \sin(\omega_0 t)\mathbf{e}_2)\ ,$$

where G and H_1 are under control. In the language of MRI, $H_0 \mathbf{e}_3$ is the static field, G the gradient, and H_1 the radio-frequency field. The input G, H_1 produces in the detecting system the output signal

$$S(t) = -\frac{d}{dt}\int_{\mathbb{R}^3} M(x, t) \cdot B(x)\,dx\ ,$$

where B characterizes the detection system. Depending on the choice of H_1, various approximations to $S(t)$ can be derived, two of which are detailed here.

Short $\pi/2$ pulse: In the first case, H_1 is constant in the small interval $[0, \tau]$ and $\gamma \int_0^\tau H_1 \, dt = \pi/2$. In that case,

$$S(t) = \int_{\mathbb{R}^3} M_0(x) e^{-i\gamma \int_0^t G(s) \, ds \cdot x - t/T_2} \, dx \ .$$

Choosing G constant for $\tau \leq t \leq \tau + T$ and zero otherwise, we get for $T << T_2$,

$$S(t) \approx (2\pi)^{3/2} \mathcal{F}(M_0)(\gamma G(t - \tau)) \ , \qquad (4.4)$$

where $\mathcal{F}(M_0)$ is the three-dimensional Fourier transform of M_0. From here we can proceed in two ways. We can use equation (4.4) to determine the three-dimensional Fourier transform $\mathcal{F}(M_0)$ of M_0 and compute M_0 by an inverse three-dimensional Fourier transform. This requires $\mathcal{F}(M_0)$ to be known on a cartesian grid, which can be achieved by a proper choice of the gradients or by interpolation. Alternatively, one can invoke the central slice theorem to obtain the three-dimensional Radon transform $R(M_0)$ of M_0 by a series of one-dimensional Fourier transforms. M_0 is then recovered by inverting the three-dimensional Radon transform.

Shaped pulse: In this case, H_1 is the shaped pulse

$$H_1(t) = \phi(t\gamma G) e^{i\gamma G x_3 t} \ ,$$

where ϕ is a smooth positive function supported in $[0, \tau]$. Then, with x', G' the first two components of x, G, respectively, we have

$$M_0'(x', x_3) = \int M_0(x', y_3) Q(x_3 - y_3) \, dy_3 \ , \qquad (4.5)$$

with a function Q essentially supported in a small neighborhood of the origin. Equation (4.5) is the two-dimensional analog of equation (4.4), and again we face the choice between Fourier imaging (*i.e.*, computing the two-dimensional Fourier transform from (4.5) and doing an inverse two-dimensional Fourier transform) and projection imaging (*i.e.*, doing a series of one-dimensional Fourier transforms on equation (4.5) and inverting the two-dimensional Radon transform).

4.2 General Issues of Image Reconstruction

We may formally state that the image reconstruction problem (or inverse problem) is finding an object function I that is consistent with the measured signal S according to a known imaging equation (or forward problem):

$$S = \mathcal{T}(I) \ ,$$

where $\mathcal{T}$ is usually an integral transformation operator. The above equation is often referred to as the data-consistency constraint, and any function satisfying this constraint is called a feasible reconstruction. The data-consistency constraint is important because image reconstruction does no more than convert information in the measured data into an image format. A violation of the data-consistency constraint can mean that this conversion step is not faithful, and a loss of valid information or a gain of spurious information may result.

If $\mathcal{T}$ is invertible, a data-consistent I can be obtained from the inverse transform such that $I = \mathcal{T}^{-1}(S)$. However, in practice, $\mathcal{T}^{-1}$ cannot be computed because the data space is only partially sampled. Therefore, instead of directly implementing the inversion formula, one focuses on finding an image function that satisfies the data-consistency constraint either by an approximate implementation of the inverse transform or by methods that may have nothing to do with it. Some general issues with such an image reconstruction procedure are existence, uniqueness, and stability.

It is easy to understand that, given a set of measured data, an object function I that is consistent with the data always exists since the data are generated from a physical object.

Whether such an object function is unique depends on how the data space is sampled. If finite sampling is used, as always the case in practice, there are many feasible object functions for a given measured data. In this case, an optimality criterion has to be applied to select an object function from the many feasible ones.

Stability of an image reconstruction technique is related to how perturbations in the data domain are translated to possible image errors. More specifically, if the data are perturbed by ΔS and, as a consequence, the image function is in error by ΔI, then $S + \Delta S = \mathcal{T}(I + \Delta I)$. An important practical question is: will ΔI be small for a small ΔS? The answer is not necessarily yes. For most imaging systems ΔS can be made negligible while ΔI is arbitrarily large. Such imaging systems are ill-conditioned and do not have a unique solution owing to finite sampling. In this case, the reconstruction problem is considered to be an ill-posed problem. Consequently, obtaining the exact true object function is theoretically impossible. However, if we pick the object function appropriately, an acceptable image can be obtained with a known deviation from true one. This deviation can be fully characterized by a point spread function (if the imaging process is linear), and it can be made negligible under certain circumstances.

4.3 Reconstruction from Fourier Transform Samples

4.3.1 Problem Formulation

For simplicity we only consider the one-dimensional case. The problem of reconstructing a function from its Fourier transform samples can be formulated as follows: Given

$$S[n] = \frac{1}{\sqrt{2\pi}} \int_{\mathbb{R}} I(x) e^{-in\Delta k\, x}\, dx, \quad n \in \mathbb{Z},$$

Δk being the fundamental frequency, determine the object function $I(x)$. It is now widely known that given a set of uniformly sampled Fourier transform samples, the discrete Fourier transform (DFT) is the computational tool to use for image reconstruction. This section discusses the basis and limitations of the DFT image reconstruction technique.

4.3.2 Basic Theory

Poisson's formula (2.9) yields

$$\sum_{n \in \mathbb{Z}} S[n] e^{in\Delta k\, x} = \frac{\sqrt{2\pi}}{\Delta k} \sum_{n \in \mathbb{Z}} I\left(x - \frac{2\pi n}{\Delta k}\right), \tag{4.6}$$

where the right-hand side is a periodic function with period $2\pi/\Delta k$.

In the remainder of this section, we derive the Fourier reconstruction formula based on (4.6). For clarity, we first discuss the infinite sampling case and then extend the result to the practical case of finite sampling.

Infinite Sampling

Suppose that $I(x)$ vanishes outside $|x| < W$, $S[n]$ is available for any $n \in \mathbb{Z}$, and $\Delta k < 2\pi/W$. Then there is no overlap among the various replicas $I(x - 2\pi n/\Delta k)$. Hence, one can obtain $I(x)$ from the Fourier series as formed in (4.6):

$$I(x) = \frac{\Delta k}{\sqrt{2\pi}} \Pi\left(\frac{\pi x}{\Delta k}\right) \sum_{n \in \mathbb{Z}} S[n] e^{in\Delta k\, x}, \tag{4.7}$$

where $\Pi(y)$ defined by

$$\Pi(y) := \chi[-1/2, 1/2](y)$$

is the rectangular window function.

Finite Sampling

Suppose that $S[n]$ is known for $-N/2 \le n < N/2$. This set is not sufficient to define the Fourier series as required by the reconstruction formula (4.7). As a result, the feasible reconstruction is not unique: If $I(x)$ is a feasible reconstruction, then $I(x) + e^{im\Delta k\, x}$ is also a feasible reconstruction for any $|m| > N/2$.

Moreover,

$$I(x) = \frac{\Delta k}{\sqrt{2\pi}} \Pi(\frac{\pi x}{\Delta k}) \left[\sum_{n=-N/2}^{N/2-1} S[n]e^{in\Delta k\, x} \right] + \sum_{n<-N/2; n\leq N/2} c_n e^{in\Delta k\, x},$$

is a feasible reconstruction for arbitrary finite c_n.

An important question regarding image reconstruction from finite Fourier transform samples is: what values should we assign to the c_n? In practice, based on the minimum-norm constraint, the unmeasured Fourier series coefficients are all forced to be zero because, according to Parseval's theorem, $\int_{-\pi/\Delta k}^{\pi/\Delta k} |I(x)|^2\, dx$ reaches the minimum when $c_n = 0$. Therefore, the minimum-norm, feasible reconstruction is in the form of a truncated Fourier series:

$$I(x) = \frac{\Delta k}{\sqrt{2\pi}} \Pi(\frac{\pi x}{\Delta k}) \sum_{n=-N/2}^{N/2-1} S[n]e^{in\Delta k\, x}, \quad |x| < \frac{\pi}{\Delta k}. \tag{4.8}$$

DFT and FFT can now be used to form an image from the continuous image function given in (4.8). Note that in spite of the discreteness of the measured data, the reconstructed image is a continuous function of space. Discretization of the image function is required by numerical computation and display.

Noise in Direct FFT Reconstruction

Suppose that N noisy data points are collected and processed using the (standard) FFT reconstruction algorithm. The image noise is given by

$$\xi_I[m] = \frac{1}{\sqrt{2\pi N}} \sum_{n=-N/2}^{N/2-1} \xi_d[n]e^{inm/N}, \quad -N/2 \leq m < N/2. \tag{4.9}$$

Several statistical properties of $\xi_I[m]$ can be directly derived from (4.9):

(i)   The image noise $\xi_I[m]$ is of zero mean, namely, $E[\xi_I[m]] = 0$.
(ii) The variance of $\xi_I[m]$ is given by $\sigma_I^2 = \sigma_d^2/\sqrt{2\pi N}$.
(iii) The image noise $\xi_I[m]$ is uncorrelated from pixel to pixel. That is to say

$$E[\xi_I[m]\overline{\xi_I[m']}] = 0 \quad \text{for } m \neq m'.$$

Moreover, by calculating the average strength per pixel I_{avg} from the Fourier reconstruction, one can see that the signal-to-noise ration per pixel $SNR|_{\text{pixel}}$ of an FFT image is inversely proportional to $\sqrt{N}$.

Specifically,

$$
\begin{aligned}
I_{\text{avg}}^2 &= \frac{1}{N} \sum_{m=-N/2}^{N/2-1} |I[m]|^2 \\
&= \frac{1}{2\pi N^3} \sum_{m=-N/2}^{N/2-1} \sum_{p=-N/2}^{N/2-1} \sum_{q=-N/2}^{N/2-1} S[p]\overline{S[q]} e^{i(p-q)m/N} \\
&= \frac{1}{2\pi N^2} \sum_{n=-N/2}^{N/2-1} |S[n]|^2 ,
\end{aligned}
$$

which yields

$$
SNR|_{\text{pixel}} = \frac{I_{\text{avg}}}{\sigma_I} = \frac{\sqrt{\sum_{n=-N/2}^{N/2-1} |S[n]|^2}}{\sqrt{N}\sigma_d} .
$$

Noting that $\sqrt{\sum_{n=-N/2}^{N/2-1} |S[n]|^2}$ stays roughly constant after N reaches a certain value, one obtains that $SNR|_{\text{pixel}}$ is inversely proportional to $\sqrt{N}$.

4.4 Reconstruction from Radon Transform Samples

Image reconstruction from Radon transform samples is commonly known as image reconstruction from projections. This problem can be formulated as follows: Given the Radon transform Rf determine f.

As in the Fourier case, if the Radon space is fully sampled, f can be uniquely determined from the inverse Radon transform formula. In practice, the Radon space is partially sampled, leading to undetermined problem. Consequently, the feasible reconstruction is not unique. Various reconstruction techniques discussed in this section represent different ways to select a reconstruction from the many feasible ones.

4.4.1 The Inverse Radon Transform

We first state some inversion formulae, which give different ways to recover a function f from its Radon transform Rf.

4.4.2 Fourier Inversion Formula

The following lemma holds.

Lemma 4.4.1 *Let* $f \in \mathcal{S}(\mathbb{R}^2)$. *Then*

$$
f(x) = \frac{1}{(2\pi)^{3/2}} \int_0^{+\infty} \tau \, d\tau \int_{S^1} e^{i\tau x \cdot \theta} \mathcal{F}(R_\theta f)(\tau) \, d\theta .
$$

Proof. We begin with the (two-dimensional) inversion formula for the Fourier transform. We have

$$f(x) = \frac{1}{2\pi} \int_{\mathbb{R}^2} e^{ix\cdot\xi} \mathcal{F}(f)(\xi)\, d\xi \ .$$

Let $\xi = \tau\theta$. Integrating in polar coordinates, we obtain that

$$f(x) = \frac{1}{2\pi} \int_0^{+\infty} \tau\, d\tau \int_{S^1} e^{i\tau x\cdot\theta} \mathcal{F}(f)(\tau\theta)\, d\theta \ .$$

We now apply the Fourier Slice Theorem to get

$$f(x) = \frac{1}{(2\pi)^{3/2}} \int_0^{+\infty} \tau\, d\tau \int_{S^1} e^{i\tau x\cdot\theta} \mathcal{F}(R_\theta f)(\tau)\, d\theta \ ,$$

as desired.   □

4.4.3 Direct Backprojection Method

To obtain another inversion formula we observe the following:

$$\int_{-\infty}^{+\infty} R_\theta f(s) g(s)\, ds = \int_{-\infty}^{+\infty} \int_{-\infty}^{+\infty} f(s\theta + t\theta^\perp) g(s)\, dt\, ds \ .$$

Let $x = s\theta + t\theta^\perp$ so that $s = x \cdot \theta$, $dx = dt\, ds$, and therefore

$$\int_{-\infty}^{+\infty} R_\theta f(s)\, g(s)\, ds = \int_{\mathbb{R}^2} f(x) g(x \cdot \theta)\, dx \ ,$$

i.e., the adjoint of R_θ is the operator $R_\theta^\star$ defined by

$$R_\theta^\star g(x) = g(x \cdot \theta) \ .$$

Consider for an arbitrary function $g(\theta, s)$, having the symmetry $g(-\theta, -s) = g(\theta, s)$. We then compute

$$\begin{aligned}
\int_{S^1 \times \mathbb{R}} Rf(\theta, s) g(\theta, s)\, d\theta\, ds &= \int_{S^1} d\theta \int_{-\infty}^{+\infty} R_\theta f(s) g(\theta, s)\, ds \\
&= \int_{S^1} d\theta \int_{-\infty}^{+\infty} f(s\theta + t\theta^\perp) g(\theta, s)\, ds\, dt \\
&= \int_{S^1} d\theta \int_{\mathbb{R}^2} f(x) g(\theta, \theta \cdot x)\, dx \\
&= \int_{\mathbb{R}^2} f(x) R^\star g(x)\, dx \ ,
\end{aligned}$$

with the definition

$$R^\star g(x) := \int_{S^1} R_\theta^\star g(x)\, d\theta \ .$$

The operator $R^\star$ is known by the name of backprojection operator. Note that $g(\theta, x)$ is a function of lines and $R^\star g$ is its integral over all lines passing through x.

The backprojection operator maps a one-dimensional profile to a two-dimensional function with constant values along a line defined by $\theta \cdot x = s$. The term backprojection comes from the fact that mapping $g(\theta, s)$ to $g(\theta, \theta \cdot x)$ is to backproject the value of $g(\theta, s_0)$ along the integration path of the Radon transform.

It is easy to prove the following useful property of the backprojection operator.

Lemma 4.4.2 Let $f \in S(\mathbb{R}^2)$ and $g \in S(\mathbb{C}^2)$. Then

$$(R^\star g) \star f = R^\star (g \star Rf) \,.$$

Finally, we get the following important result, which plays an important role in the numerical inversion of the Radon transform. It is the starting point for the filtered backprojection algorithm.

Lemma 4.4.3 Let $f \in S(\mathbb{R}^2)$. Then

$$R^\star Rf = \frac{2}{|x|} \star f \,.$$

Proof.   We have

$$R^\star Rf = \int_{S^1} Rf(\theta, \theta \cdot x) \, d\theta$$

$$= \int_{S^1} d\theta \int_{-\infty}^{+\infty} f((\theta \cdot x)\theta + s\theta^\perp) \, ds$$

$$= \int_{S^1} d\theta \int_{-\infty}^{+\infty} f(x + s\theta^\perp) \, ds$$

$$= 2 \int_{S^1} d\theta \int_0^{+\infty} f(x + s\theta^\perp) \, ds \,.$$

By setting $y = s\theta^\perp, s = |y|, dy = s \, d\theta \, ds$, we get

$$R^\star Rf = 2 \int_{\mathbb{R}^2} \frac{1}{|y|} f(x + y) \, dy$$

$$= 2 \int_{\mathbb{R}^2} \frac{1}{|x - y|} f(y) \, dy \,,$$

as desired.   □

From $\mathcal{F}(1/|y|) = 1/(2\pi|\xi|)$, it follows that

$$\mathcal{F}(R^\star Rf)(\xi) = \frac{2}{|\xi|} \mathcal{F}(f)(\xi) \,.$$

Therefore, we can conclude that the inversion operator Λ is such that

$$\mathcal{F}^{-1}(\Lambda) = |\xi|/2$$

so that

$$f(x) = \frac{1}{4\pi} \int_{\mathbb{R}^2} e^{ix\cdot\xi} |\xi| \mathcal{F}(R^\star Rf)(\xi) \, d\xi = \Lambda R^\star Rf(x) \, . \qquad (4.10)$$

Formula (4.10) is called the backprojection inversion formula.

Formula (4.10) is the general backprojection reconstruction formula where the measured projection profiles are first backpropagated and then integrated over the unit disk. The point spread function associated with backprojection reconstruction is $1/|x|$.

In practice, the measured projections are discretized both angularly and radially. We may assume that $Rf(\theta, p)$ is available at the following points:

$$\theta = \theta_{n_\theta} = (\cos(n_\theta \Delta\theta), \sin(n_\theta \Delta\theta)), \quad n_\theta = 0, 1, \ldots, N_\theta - 1 \, ,$$
$$p = p_{n_p} = n_p \Delta p, \quad n_p = -N_p/2, \ldots, N_p/2 - 1 \, .$$

Then,

$$f(x) = \Lambda R^\star \left[\Delta\theta \sum_{n_\theta=0}^{N_\theta - 1} Rf(\theta_{n_\theta}, p_{n_p}) \right](x) \, .$$

A notable limitation of the backprojection method is that it produces blurred images. This problem can be overcome using the filtered backprojection reconstruction method.

4.4.4 Filtered Backprojection Reconstruction

Filtered backprojection reconstruction is a direct implementation of the inverse Radon transform formula. It differs from the direct backprojection reconstruction only in that measured projections are filtered before they are backpropagated.

Let the Hilbert transform H be defined by

$$Hg(s) = \frac{1}{\pi} \text{p.v.} \int_{-\infty}^{+\infty} \frac{g(t)}{s - t} dt \, .$$

Here p.v. means the Cauchy principal value. The filtered backprojection inversion formula reads

$$f = \frac{1}{4\pi} R^\star H(Rf)' ,$$

where

$$(Rf)'(\theta, s) = (\frac{\partial}{\partial s} R_\theta f)(s) \, .$$

In other words,

$$f(x) = \frac{1}{(2\pi)^2} \int_{S^1} \int_{\mathbb{R}} \frac{(Rf)'(\theta, t)}{x \cdot \theta - t} \, dt \, d\theta \ .$$

An approximate implementation of this formula can be given using the Fourier inversion formula

$$f(x) \approx \int_0^\pi Q(x \cdot \theta) \, dt \ ,$$

where, $\theta = (\cos t, \sin t)$, and

$$Q(t) = \frac{1}{\sqrt{2\pi}} \int_{-b}^{b} |\tau| e^{it\tau} \mathcal{F}(Rf)(\tau) \, d\tau$$

$$\approx \frac{1}{\sqrt{2\pi}} \int_{-\infty}^{+\infty} |\tau| e^{it\tau} \mathcal{F}(Rf)(\tau) \, d\tau \ .$$

This last approximation constitutes a band limiting process, where the used filter function is known by the name of Ram-Lak filter. Indeed, to limit the unbounded nature of the $|\tau|$ filter in the high-frequency range, which amplifies high-frequency noise, we can multiply it with a bandlimiting function such as the rectangular window function $\Pi(\tau/b)$, where $\Pi(x) = \chi([-1, 1])$. Other filter functions such as the generalized Hamming filter

$$G_b(\tau) := |\tau| H(2\pi \frac{\tau}{b}) \Pi(\frac{\tau}{b}) \ ,$$

H being defined by (2.23), the Shepp-Logan filter or the low-pass cosine filter can be used and yield noticeably different reconstructions.

4.4.5 Noise in Filtered Backprojection Reconstruction

Consider the filtered backprojection reconstruction. Let $\xi_d[n_p, n_\theta]$ be the additive noise in a polar data set consisting of N_θ radial lines, each with N_p points. Then, the image noise from filtered backprojection is given by

$$\xi_I[x] = \frac{\pi}{\sqrt{2\pi} N_\theta N_p} \sum_{n_\theta=0}^{N_\theta-1} \sum_{n_p=-N_p/2}^{N_p/2-1} \frac{|n_p|}{N_p} \xi_d[n_p, n_\theta] e^{i n_p n_\theta} \ .$$

Based on this equation, it is easy to show that

$$E[\xi_I[x]] = 0 \quad \text{if} \quad E[\xi_d[n_p, n_\theta]] = 0 \ .$$

In other words, the image noise has a zero mean if the mean of the data noise is zero, as is the often the case in practice.

To derive the image noise variance, we further assume that $\xi_d[p_{n_p}, \theta_{n_\theta}]$ is uncorrelated from one measurement to another.

Under this assumption, we have

$$\text{var}[\xi_I[x]] = \frac{\pi}{2}\left(\frac{1}{N_\theta N_p}\right)^2 \sum_{n_\theta=0}^{N_\theta-1} \sum_{n_p=-N_p/2}^{N_p/2-1} (\frac{n_p}{N_p})^2 \text{var}[\xi_d[n_p,n_\theta]] \,.$$

With the notation $\text{var}[\xi_I] = \sigma_I^2[FBP]$ and $\text{var}[\xi_d] = \sigma_d^2$, we have

$$\sigma_I^2[FBP] = \left(\frac{\pi}{N_\theta N_p}\right)^2 \sum_{n_\theta=0}^{N_\theta-1} \sum_{n_p=-N_p/2}^{N_p/2-1} (\frac{n_p}{N_p})^2 \sigma_d^2$$

$$\approx \frac{\pi}{24 N_\theta N_p}\sigma_d^2 \,,$$

where $\sum_{n=0}^{N} n^2 = (1/6)\,N(N+1)(2N+1) \approx (1/3)\,N^3$ is used.

Note that for two-dimensional Fourier imaging with $N_p \times N_\theta$ Cartesian points, we have

$$\sigma_I^2[FT] = \frac{1}{2\pi N_p^2 N_\theta^2} \sum_{n_p=-N_p/2-1}^{N_p/2} \sum_{n_\theta=-N_\theta/2}^{N_\theta/2-1} \text{var}[\xi_d[n_p,n_\theta]]$$

$$= \frac{1}{2\pi N_p N_\theta}\sigma_d^2 \,.$$

Therefore,

$$\frac{\sigma_I[FBP]}{\sigma_I[FT]} \approx \frac{\pi}{\sqrt{12}} \,.$$

Bibliography and Discussion

An excellent reference on tomographic imaging with non-diffracting sources is the book by Natterer and Wübbeling [103]. In particular, this book provides readers with a superior understanding of the mathematical methods in computerized tomographic imaging and more advanced topics, such as the attenuated Radon transform and the helical CT.

5

Tomographic Imaging with Diffracting Sources

Tomographic imaging with diffracting sources can be modelled as inverse problems for partial differential equations. Linearized versions lead to problems similar to those in tomographic imaging with non-diffracting sources, except that the straight lines are replaced by more complex shapes. In this chapter, we single out three non-ionizing imaging methods: (i) electrical impedance tomography; (ii) ultrasound imaging, and (iii) microwave imaging. These three techniques form an important alternative to straight ray tomography (CT) and MRI. In ultrasound and microwave imaging modalities, the interaction of a field and an object is modelled with the Helmholtz equation while in EIT, the mathematical model reduces to the conductivity equation. One general reconstruction algorithm used in ultrasound and microwave imaging is the diffraction tomography.

For some applications, the harm caused by the use of X-rays, an ionizing radiation, could outweigh any benefits that might be gained from the tomogram. This is one reason for the interest in imaging with electric, acoustic, or electromagnetic radiation, which are considered safe at low levels. In addition, these modalities measure the electrical, acoustic, and electromagnetic properties of tissues and thus make available information that is not obtainable from X-ray tomography or MRI images. Thirdly, they are easily portable and relatively inexpensive.

In this chapter we first describe general algorithms used in electrical impedance tomography. Then we present the mathematical basis of diffraction tomography.

5.1 Electrical Impedance Tomography

There are a variety of medical problems for which it would be useful to know the distribution of the electrical properties inside the body. By electrical properties we mean specifically the electric conductivity and permittivity. The electric conductivity is a measure of the ease with which a material conducts electricity; the electric permittivity is a measure of how readily the charges within a material separate under an imposed electric field. Both of these properties are of interest in medical applications, because different tissues have different conductivities and permittivities.

One important medical problem for which knowledge of internal electrical properties would be useful is the detection of breast cancer.

In this section we present the mathematical model for EIT. We use this model to describe some reconstruction algorithms.

5.1.1 Mathematical Model

The electric potential or voltage u in the body Ω is governed by the conductivity equation

$$\nabla \cdot \gamma(x,\omega)\nabla u = 0, \quad x \in \Omega . \tag{5.1}$$

Here γ is given by $\gamma(x,\omega) = \sigma(x,\omega) + i\omega\varepsilon(x,\omega)$, where σ is the electric conductivity, ε is the electric permittivity, and ω is the angular frequency of the applied current.

In practice, we apply currents to electrodes on the surface $\partial\Omega$ of the body. These currents produce a current density on the surface whose inward pointing normal component is denoted by g. Thus,

$$\gamma\frac{\partial u}{\partial\nu} = g \quad \text{on } \partial\Omega . \tag{5.2}$$

The mathematical model of EIT is (5.1) and (5.2), together with the conservation of charge condition $\int_{\partial\Omega} g = 0$ and the condition $\int_{\partial\Omega} u = 0$, which amounts to choosing a reference voltage. The injected currents can be approximated by linear combinations of dipoles. A dipole at a point $z \in \partial\Omega$ is given by $-|\partial\Omega|\, \partial\delta_z/\partial T$, $\partial/\partial T$ being the tangential derivative at $\partial\Omega$. The operator $g \mapsto u|_{\partial\Omega}$ is called the Neumann-to-Dirichlet boundary map.

The reconstruction problem in EIT is to obtain an approximation of γ in Ω from the boundary measurements of u on $\partial\Omega$. This problem is challenging because it is not only nonlinear, but also severely ill-posed, which means that large changes in the interior can correspond to very small changes in the measured data.

From a theoretical point of view, all possible boundary measurements uniquely determine γ in Ω. However, in practice we are limited to a finite number of current-to-voltage patterns.

Before describing classical reconstruction algorithms in EIT, we explain the fundamental shortcomings of EIT in detail by use of its discretized version.

5.1.2 Ill-Conditioning

For simplicity, we suppose that Ω is a square region in $\mathbb{R}^2$. We divide Ω uniformly into $N \times N$ sub-squares Ω_{ij} with the center point (x_i, y_j), where

$i, j = 0, \ldots, N - 1$. The goal of EIT is to determine $N \times N$ conductivity values under the assumption that the conductivity γ is constant on each subsquare Ω_{ij}, say γ_{ij}. Let

$$\Sigma = \left\{ \gamma : \gamma|_{\Omega_{ij}} = \text{constant for } i, j = 0, \ldots, N - 1 \right\}.$$

For a given $\gamma \in \Sigma$, the solution u of the direct problem (5.1) and (5.2) can be approximated by a vector $U = (u_0, u_1, \ldots, u_{N^2-1})$ such that each interior voltage $u_k, k = i + jN$ is determined by the weighted average (depending on γ) of the four neighboring potentials. More precisely, a discretized form of (5.1) is given by

$$u_k = \frac{1}{a_{kk}} \left[a_{kk_N} u_{k_N} + a_{kk_S} u_{k_S} + a_{kk_E} u_{k_E} + a_{kk_W} u_{k_W} \right],$$

with

$$a_{kk} = -\sum_l a_{kk_l} \quad \text{and} \quad a_{kk_l} = \frac{\gamma_k \gamma_l}{\gamma_k + \gamma_l} \quad \text{for } l = N, S, E, W.$$

Here k_N, k_S, k_E, k_W denote north, south, east, and west neighboring of k-th point. The discretized conductivity equation (5.1) with the Neumann boundary condition (5.2) can be written as a linear system $A_\gamma U = G$, where G is the injection current vector associated with g. Let F denote the small-size sub-vector of U restricted to $\partial\Omega$, which corresponds to the boundary voltage potential on $\partial\Omega$. Then the inverse conductivity problem is to determine γ, or equivalently A_γ, from one or several measurements of current-to-voltage pairs $(G^m, F^m), m = 1, \ldots, M$.

The fundamental shortcoming of EIT for providing high resolution images is due to the fact that reconstructing A_γ from $(G^m, F^m), m = 1, \ldots, M$, is exponentially difficult as the matrix size A_γ increases. More precisely, the value of the potential at each Ω_{ij} inside Ω can be expressed as the weighted average of its neighboring potentials where weights are determined by the conductivity distribution. Therefore, the measured data F is entangled in the global structure of the conductivity distribution in a highly nonlinear way and any internal conductivity value γ_{ij} has a little influence on boundary measurements if Ω_{ij} is away from the boundary. This phenomenon causes the ill-posedness nature of EIT.

5.1.3 Static Imaging

Static image reconstruction problem is based on iterative methods. An image reconstruction algorithm iteratively updates the conductivity distribution until it minimizes in the least-squares sense the difference between measured data and computed boundary voltages. As part of each iteration in the minimization, a forward solver is used to determine the boundary voltages that would be produced given the applied currents. This technique was first introduced in EIT by Yorkey, Webster, and Tompkins in the 80's following a number of variations and improvements. These include utilization of a priori information, various forms of regularization, and adaptive mesh refinement. Even though this approach is widely adopted for static imaging by many researchers, it requires a large amount of computation time for producing static images even with low spatial resolution and poor accuracy.

Because of the fundamental limitations of EIT, it seems from a practical point of view reasonable to restrict ourselves to find the deviation of the conductivity from an assumedly known conductivity.

5.1.4 Dynamic Imaging

The algorithms described here are based on approximations to the linearized EIT problem.

Barber-Brown Backprojection Algorithm

The Barber-Brown Backprojection algorithm is the first fast and useful algorithm in EIT although it provides images with very low resolution. It is based on the assumption that the conductivity does not differ very much from a constant and can be viewed as a generalized Radon transform.

For simplicity, suppose that Ω is the unit disk in $\mathbb{R}^2$ and γ is a small perturbation of a constant $\gamma = \gamma_0 + \delta\gamma$ in Ω. In the simplest case we assume $\gamma_0 = 1$, so that

$$\gamma(x) = 1 + \delta\gamma(x), \quad |\delta\gamma(x)| << 1, x \in \Omega , \tag{5.3}$$

and we further assume that $\delta\gamma = 0$ on $\partial\Omega$. Let u_0 and u denote the potentials corresponding to γ_0 and γ with the same Neumann boundary data $g = -2\pi\partial\delta_z/\partial\theta$ at a point $z \in \partial\Omega$. Writing $u = u_0 + \delta u$, δu satisfies approximately the equation

$$-\Delta\delta u \approx \nabla\delta\gamma \cdot \nabla u_0 \quad \text{in } \Omega , \tag{5.4}$$

with the homogeneous boundary condition. Here, the term $\nabla\delta\gamma \cdot \nabla\delta u$ is neglected.

Observe that

$$u_0(x) = \frac{x \cdot z^\perp}{|x - z|^2} ,$$

where $z^\perp$ is the rotate of z by $\pi/2$. Next, we introduce a holomorphic function in Ω whose real part is $-u_0$:

$$\Psi_z(x) := s + it := -\frac{x \cdot z^\perp}{|x - z|^2} + i\frac{1 - z \cdot x}{|x - z|^2} .$$

Then we can view Ψ_z as a transform which maps the unit disk Ω onto the upper half plane $\widetilde{\Omega} := \{s + it : t > 1/2\}$. Hence, we can view x as a function with respect to $\Psi_z = s + it$ defined in $\widetilde{\Omega}$. Let $\widetilde{\delta u}_z(\Psi_z(x)) = \delta u(x)$ and $\widetilde{\delta \gamma}(\Psi_z(x)) = \delta\gamma(x)$. Using the fact that $\nabla s \cdot \nabla t = 0$ and $|\nabla s| = |\nabla t|$, it follows from (5.4) that

$$
\begin{cases}
\Delta \widetilde{\delta u} = -\dfrac{\partial \widetilde{\delta\gamma}}{\partial s} & \text{in } \widetilde{\Omega} , \\[2mm]
\left. \dfrac{\partial \widetilde{\delta u}}{\partial t} \right|_{t=1/2} = 0 .
\end{cases}
$$

Hence, if $\widetilde{\delta\gamma}$ is independent of the t–variable, $\widetilde{\delta u}$ depends only on s and $\widetilde{\delta\gamma}$. With the notation $z = (\cos\theta, \sin\theta)$, Barber and Brown derived from this idea the following reconstruction formula:

$$
\delta\gamma(x) = \widetilde{\delta\gamma}(\Psi_z(x)) = \frac{1}{2\pi} \int_0^{2\pi} \frac{\partial}{\partial s} \widetilde{\delta u}_z\left(s + \frac{i}{2}\right) d\theta .
$$

Dynamic Imaging

Suppose that currents $g^n, n = 1, \ldots, N$, are applied on $\partial\Omega$. Application of g^n gives rise to the potential u^n inside Ω. In dynamic imaging, we measure the boundary voltage potential $f^n = u^n|_\Omega$ to reconstruct the change of the conductivity $\delta\gamma$ from the relation between g^n and f^n. Let u_0^n denote the background potential, that is, the solution to

$$
\begin{cases}
\Delta u_0^n = 0 & \text{in } \Omega , \\[2mm]
\dfrac{\partial u_0^n}{\partial \nu} = g^n & \text{on } \partial\Omega , \\[2mm]
\int_{\partial\Omega} u_0^n = 0 .
\end{cases}
$$

Set $\delta u^n = u^n - u_0^n$. The reconstruction algorithm is based on the following identity

$$
\int_\Omega \delta\gamma \nabla u_0^n \cdot \nabla u_0^m = \int_{\partial\Omega} (g^n f_0^m - f^n g^m) - \int_\Omega \delta\gamma \nabla \delta u^n \cdot \nabla u_0^m .
$$

Since the last term in the above identity can be regarded as negligibly small, the perturbation $\delta\gamma$ can be computed from

$$
\int_\Omega \delta\gamma \nabla u_0^n \cdot \nabla u_0^m = b[n, m] ,
$$

where $b[n, m] = \int_{\partial\Omega} (g^n f_0^m - f^n g^m)$.

5.1.5 Electrode Model

The continuum model (5.1) and (5.2) is a poor model for real experiments, because we do not know the current density g. In practice, we know only the currents that are sent down wires attached to discrete electrodes, which in turn are attached to the body. One might approximate the unknown current density as a constant over each electrode, but this model also turns out to be inadequate. We need to account for two main effects: the discreteness of the electrodes, and the extra conductive material (the electrodes themselves) we have added. We should account for the electrochemical effect that takes place at the contact between the electrode and the body. This effect is the formation of a thin, highly resistive layer between the electrode and the body. The impedance of this layer is characterized by a number z_n, called the effective contact impedance. See Fig. 5.1 for a prototype EIT probe.

Let e_n denote the part of $\partial\Omega$ that corresponds to the nth electrode and let I_n be the current sent to the electrode e_n. The electrode model consists of (5.1),

$$\int_{e_n} \gamma \frac{\partial u}{\partial \nu} = I_n, \quad n = 1, \ldots, N ,$$

$$\gamma \frac{\partial u}{\partial \nu} = 0 \quad \text{in the gap between the electrodes,}$$

the constraint

$$u + z_n \gamma \frac{\partial u}{\partial \nu} = V_n \quad \text{on } e_n, \quad n = 1, \ldots, N ,$$

where V_n, for $n = 1, \ldots, N$, is the measured potential on the electrode e_n and z_n is the contact impedance assumed to be known, together with the conditions

$$\sum_{n=1}^{N} I_n = 0 \quad \text{(conservation of charge)}$$

and

$$\sum_{n=1}^{N} V_n = 0 \quad \text{(choice of a ground).}$$

This model has been shown to have a unique solution and able to predict the experimental measurements.

5.2 Ultrasound and Microwave Tomographies

Propagation of acoustical and electromagnetic waves in biological tissue is described by linear wave equations. Although the physical interpretation varies, these equations largely coincide. Ultrasound and microwave tomographies can be done in the time domain and the frequency domain. A standard inversion technique in ultrasound and microwave imaging in the frequency domain is the diffraction tomography.

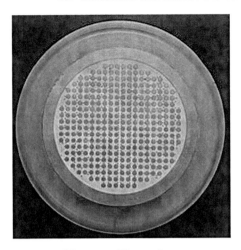

Fig. 5.1. Electrodes.

5.2.1 Mathematical Model

In ultrasound and microwave imaging, the object to be imaged is irradiated by a plane wave $u_I(x) = e^{i\omega x \cdot \theta}$, with the wavelength $\lambda := 2\pi/\omega$, travelling in the direction of the unit vector θ. The relevant equation is the Helmholtz equation

$$\Delta u + \omega^2 (1 + q)u = 0 \quad \text{in } \mathbb{R}^d ,$$

subject to the Sommerfeld radiation condition on the scattered field $u_S := u - u_I$ at infinity, where the object is given by the function q, which vanishes outside the object. The total field u is measured outside the object for many directions θ. From all these measurements, the function q has to be determined.

The scattered field u_S satisfies the Sommerfeld radiation condition and the Helmholtz equation

$$\Delta u_S + \omega^2 u_S = -\omega^2 (u_I + u_S)q . \tag{5.5}$$

Now we assume that the function q is supported in $|x| < \rho$ and $|q| << 1$. Then we can neglect u_S on the right-hand side of (5.5), obtaining

$$\Delta u_S + \omega^2 u_S \approx -\omega^2 u_I q .$$

This equation can be solved for u_S with the help of the outgoing Green function Γ_ω for the Helmholtz operator $\Delta + \omega^2$. We have the so-called Born approximation

$$u_S(x) \approx -\omega^2 \int_{|y|<\rho} \Gamma_\omega(x - y) e^{i\omega\theta \cdot y} q(y) \, dy . \tag{5.6}$$

Note that problem (5.5) is a regularly perturbed problem, and therefore, neglecting u_S on the right-hand side of (5.5) can be fully justified.

5.2.2 Diffraction Tomography

In diffraction tomography, one computes for weakly scattering objects the Fourier transform of the object function from the Fourier transform of the measured scattered data.

To present the basics of diffraction tomography, we first recall that the Green function Γ_ω has the plane wave decomposition

$$\Gamma_\omega(x) = -ic_d \int_{\mathbb{R}^{d-1}} \frac{1}{\beta} e^{i(\beta|x_d|+\alpha\cdot\tilde{x})} \, d\alpha, \quad x = (\tilde{x}, x_d), \tilde{x} = (x_1, \ldots, x_{d-1}),$$

where

$$\beta = \begin{cases} \sqrt{\omega^2 - |\alpha|^2}, & |\alpha| < \omega, \\ i\sqrt{|\alpha|^2 - \omega^2}, & |\alpha| \geq \omega, \end{cases}$$

and

$$c_2 = \frac{1}{4\pi}, \quad c_3 = \frac{1}{8\pi^2}.$$

Substituting this expression into the Born approximation (5.6) for the scattered field u_S yields

$$u_S(x) \approx i\omega^2 c_d \int_{\mathbb{R}^{d-1}} \int_{|y|<\rho} \frac{q(y)}{\beta} e^{i(\beta|x_d-y_d|+\alpha\cdot(\tilde{x}-\tilde{y}))} e^{i\omega\theta\cdot y} \, dy \, d\alpha, \qquad (5.7)$$

where $y = (\tilde{y}, y_d)$.

Suppose for simplicity that $d = 2$, $\theta = (0,1)$, and u, hence u_S, is measured on the line $x_2 = l$, where l is greater than any y_2-coordinate within the object. Then (5.7) may be rewritten as

$$u_S(x_1, l) \approx \frac{i\omega^2}{4\pi} \int_{-\infty}^{+\infty} d\alpha \int_{|y|<\rho} \frac{q(y)}{\beta} e^{i(\beta(l-y_2)+\alpha\cdot(x_1-y_1))} e^{i\omega y_2} \, dy.$$

Recognizing part of the inner integral as the two-dimensional Fourier transform of the object function q evaluated at $(\alpha, \beta - \omega)$ we find

$$u_S(x_1, l) \approx \frac{i\omega^2}{2} \int_{-\infty}^{+\infty} \frac{1}{\beta} e^{i(\beta l + \alpha x_1)} \mathcal{F}(q)(\alpha, \beta - \omega) \, d\alpha.$$

Taking the one-dimensional Fourier transform of $u_S(x_1, l)$, we obtain

$$\mathcal{F}(u_S(\cdot, l))(\alpha) \approx i\omega^2 \sqrt{\frac{\pi}{2}} \frac{1}{\sqrt{\omega^2 - \alpha^2}} e^{i\sqrt{\omega^2-\alpha^2}l} \mathcal{F}(q)(\alpha, \sqrt{\omega^2 - \alpha^2} - \omega)$$

for $|\alpha| < \omega$.

This expression relates the two-dimensional Fourier transform of the object function to the one-dimensional Fourier transform of the scattered field at the receiver line $x_2 = l$.

The factor

$$i\omega^2 \sqrt{\frac{\pi}{2}} \frac{1}{\sqrt{\omega^2 - \alpha^2}} e^{i\sqrt{\omega^2 - \alpha^2}l}$$

is a simple constant for a fixed receiver line and operating frequency ω. As α varies from $-\omega$ to ω, the coordinates $(\alpha, \sqrt{\omega^2 - \alpha^2} - \omega)$ in the Fourier transform of q trace out a semicircular arc. The endpoints of this semicircular arc are at the distance $\sqrt{2}\,\omega$ from the origin in the Fourier domain. Therefore, if the object is illuminated from many different θ-directions, we can fill up a disk of diameter $\sqrt{2}\,\omega$ in the Fourier domain and then reconstruct the object function $q(x)$ by direct Fourier inversion. The reconstructed object is a low pass version of the original one.

Bibliography and Discussion

Static image reconstruction problem in EIT was first considered in [126, 124]. The backprojection algorithm was introduced by Barber and Brown in [25]. Santosa and Vogelius [111] recognized explicitly that some sort of Radon transform was involved in backprojection. Dynamic imaging in EIT has been developed by Isaacson's group [71, 69, 70, 62, 41, 40, 42]. The electrode model was investigated in [117]. Kaczmarz's method can be applied for solving the nonlinear problem in EIT [103].

An important problem in EIT is to decide, what the optimal, or most informative measurement setting. This problem is referred to as the optimal current pattern problem. It was proved in [62] that the optimal current pattern is the eigenvalue corresponding to the maximal eigenvalue (in absolute value) of the difference between the Neumann-to-Dirichlet boundary map associated with the true conductivity and the one associated with an *a priori* estimate of it.

The reader is referred to Devaney [49] for diffraction tomography. A very promising inversion approach in ultrasound in the time domain is the time-reversal technique. This technique has been largely developed by Fink's group at LOA [56]. See Sect. 8.3.

For solving inverse problems in EIT and ultrasound imaging, it is important to have fast and reliable algorithms for the forward problems. Such algorithms are available for EIT, since algorithms for the conductivity equation are a well-established field in numerical analysis. For ultrasound, one has to solve Helmholtz-type equations at high frequencies, which still is a challenge.

One of the most challenging problems in EIT is that in practical measurements, one usually lacks exact knowledge of the boundary of the domain Ω. Because of this, the numerical reconstruction from the measured EIT data is done using a model domain that represents the best guess for the true domain. However, it has been noticed that an inaccurate model of the boundary causes severe errors for the reconstructions. An elegant and original solution toward eliminating the error caused by an incorrectly modeled boundary in EIT has been proposed and implemented numerically in [84].

6

Biomagnetic Source Imaging

The human brain is a complicated inhomogeneous and anisotropic conductor (with conductivity showing directional dependence) within which primary currents of electrochemical origin are generated. All this electromagnetic activity of the brain gives rise to electric and magnetic fields which can be measured outside the head with very sophisticated and sensitive equipments. Given the electromagnetic activity of the brain as well as its physical and geometrical characteristics we can calculate the electric and/or the magnetic field outside the head. This forms the forward electric or magnetic problem for the brain. From the point of view of medical diagnosis though the importance lies with the corresponding inverse problems, where we seek algorithms to recover the activity of the sources that produced these fields.

Electroencephalography (EEG) and magnetoencephalography (MEG) are two complementary non-invasive imaging modalities based, respectively, on the measurement of the electric potential on the scalp (EEG), and of the magnetic flux density 6-7 cm away from the head (MEG) produced by neural current sources within the brain. Clinical applications of EEG and MEG include improved understanding and treatment of serious neurological and neuropsychological disorders such as epilepsy, depression, and Parkinson's and Alzheimer's diseases.

The reconstruction of the underlying sources in EEG and MEG is a severely ill-posed inverse problem. Most approaches used to solve the source estimation problem can be roughly classified as either imaging or parametric source models. Imaging relies on assigning an element current source to each area element of the cortex, and solving the resulting inverse problem. This produces a highly under-determined problem, the regularization of it leads to over-smoothed current distributions. An alternative approach is using a parametric representation for the neural source. Such methods include the equivalent current dipole (ECD), its extension to multiple current dipole models, and the multiple expansion methods which adequately describe sources with significant spatial extent and arbitrary activation patterns.

In this chapter, we only consider the ECD model which is adequate to describe realistic generators of focal human brain activity. Such focal brain activation can be observed in epilepsy, or it can be induced by a stimulus in neurophysiological or neuropsychological experiments. We review basic results on EEG and MEG for a spherical model of the brain.

6.1 Mathematical Models

Given a set of MEG or EEG signals from an array of external sensors, the inverse problem involves estimation of the properties of the current sources within the brain that produced these signals. Before we can make such an estimate, we must first understand and solve the forward problem, in which we compute the scalp potentials and external electromagnetic fields for a specific set of neural current sources.

Let us begin with the introduction of some notation: let $\mathbf{E}$ be the electric field, $\mathbf{B}$ the magnetic induction, μ the magnetic permeability. We assume that μ is constant over the whole volume and is equal to the permeability of vacuum.

In the considered low-frequency band (frequencies below 1 kHz for the electromagnetic waves in the brain), the quasi-static theory of electromagnetism is adequate to study the brain activity. This approximation ignores the temporal variations of the electric and the magnetic fields, and therefore it eliminates the wave character of the theory. Nevertheless, it is not a static theory since it allows for current flows. Therefore, the governing equations, called the quasi-static Maxwell equations in $\mathbb{R}^3$, read as

$$\begin{cases} \nabla \times \mathbf{E} = 0, \quad \nabla \cdot \mathbf{E} = 0 \,, \\ \nabla \times \mathbf{B} = \mu \mathbf{J}, \quad \nabla \cdot \mathbf{B} = 0 \,, \end{cases} \tag{6.1}$$

where

$$\mathbf{J} = \mathbf{J}^P + \gamma \mathbf{E}$$

is the total current which is the superposition of the neural current (the so-called primary or impressed current) $\mathbf{J}^P$, *i.e.,* the current that is electrochemically generated in the neurons, and the secondary or induction current, $\gamma \mathbf{E}$, which is due to the conductivity of the brain tissues, the cerebrospinal fluid, the bones of the skull and the scalp. The induction current is proportional to the electric field.

Let Ω denote the head domain. We suppose that Ω is a simply connected smooth domain and $\mathbf{J}^P$ is compactly supported in Ω.

For a homogeneous model of the head system γ is constant in the head and $\gamma = 0$ outside the head. The irrotationality of the electric field $\mathbf{E}$ implies that there exists a scalar function u, called the voltage potential, such that

$$\mathbf{E} = -\nabla u \quad \text{in } \mathbb{R}^3 \,.$$

Therefore, from (6.1) it follows that

$$\frac{1}{\mu}\nabla \times \mathbf{B} = \mathbf{J}^P - \gamma\nabla u \quad \text{in } \mathbb{R}^3 \ . \tag{6.2}$$

6.1.1 The Electric Forward Problem

Taking the divergence of equation (6.2) gives the equation

$$\gamma\Delta u = \nabla \cdot \mathbf{J}^P \quad \text{in } \Omega \ , \tag{6.3}$$

which describes the potential distribution in the head domain Ω due to a primary current $\mathbf{J}^P$ in the brain. For the electric forward problem, the primary current and the conductivity are known, and the equation has to be solved for the unknown potential u with the homogeneous Neumann boundary condition on the head surface,

$$\frac{\partial u}{\partial \nu} = 0 \quad \text{on } \partial\Omega \ .$$

Additionally, $\int_{\partial\Omega} u = 0$.

Using the ECD model, $\mathbf{J}^P = \sum_{s=1}^m \mathbf{q}_s \delta_{z_s}$, where m is the number of sources, $\mathbf{q}_s$ the dipolar moment of the source s and $z_s \in \Omega$ its location. The corresponding source term in equation (6.3) is $\sum_{s=1}^m \mathbf{q}_s \cdot \nabla\delta_{z_s}$, which yields the potential

$$u(x) = \frac{1}{\gamma}\sum_{s=1}^m \mathbf{q}_s \cdot \nabla N(x, z_s) \ , \tag{6.4}$$

where N is the Neumann function given by (3.22).

6.1.2 The Magnetic Forward Problem

Since the divergence of $\mathbf{B}$ is zero, a magnetic potential $\mathbf{A}$ with $\mathbf{B} = \nabla \times \mathbf{A}$ can be introduced and, using Coulomb's gauge $\nabla \cdot \mathbf{A} = 0$, the quasi-static Maxwell equations (6.1) transform to

$$\nabla\nabla\mathbf{A} = -\Delta\mathbf{A} + \nabla\nabla \cdot \mathbf{A} = -\Delta\mathbf{A} = \mu(\mathbf{J}^P - \gamma\nabla u) \quad \text{in } \mathbb{R}^3 \ .$$

Since the source term is vanishing outside Ω, $\mathbf{A}$ is given by

$$\mathbf{A} = \frac{\mu}{4\pi}\int_\Omega \frac{\mathbf{J}^P(y) - \gamma\nabla u(y)}{|x - y|} \, dy \ .$$

Therefore,

$$\mathbf{B}(x) = \frac{\mu}{4\pi}\int_\Omega \mathbf{J}(y) \times \frac{x - y}{|x - y|^3} \, dy \ , \tag{6.5}$$

which is the Biot-Savart law of magnetism.

Inserting the expression

$$\mathbf{J}(y) = \sum_{s=1}^{m} \mathbf{q}_s \delta_{z_s} - \gamma \nabla u(y)$$

in the equation (6.5) we obtain

$$\mathbf{B}(x) = \frac{\mu}{4\pi} \sum_{s=1}^{m} \mathbf{q}_s \times \frac{x - z_s}{|x - z_s|^3} - \frac{\mu\gamma}{4\pi} \int_{\Omega} \nabla u(y) \times \frac{x - y}{|x - y|^3} \, dy \,. \qquad (6.6)$$

Since

$$\nabla_y u(y) \times \frac{x - y}{|x - y|^3} = \nabla_y \times \left(u(y) \frac{x - y}{|x - y|^3} \right),$$

and, by integrating by parts,

$$\int_{\Omega} \nabla_y \times \left(u(y) \frac{x - y}{|x - y|^3} \right) dy = \int_{\partial\Omega} u(y)\nu(y) \times \frac{x - y}{|x - y|^3} \, d\sigma(y) \,,$$

equation (6.5) can be transformed into Geselowitz formula

$$\mathbf{B}(x) = \frac{\mu}{4\pi} \sum_{s=1}^{m} \mathbf{q}_s \times \frac{x - z_s}{|x - z_s|^3} - \frac{\mu\gamma}{4\pi} \int_{\partial\Omega} u(y)\nu(y) \times \frac{x - y}{|x - y|^3} d\sigma(y) \,. \qquad (6.7)$$

The physical interpretation of the representation formula (6.7) is the following. The first term on the right-hand side represents the contribution of the primary current dipoles while the integral represents the contribution of the conductive medium. In formula (6.6) the conductive medium behaves as a volume distribution of electric dipoles with moments equal to $-\gamma\nabla u$, while formula (6.7) shows that this distribution can be also interpreted as an equivalent surface distribution of dipoles over the boundary $\partial\Omega$ with moments $-\gamma u\,\nu$ normal to the boundary. Therefore, the exterior magnetic field $\mathbf{B}$ is strongly dependent on the geometry of the conductive medium.

6.2 The Inverse EEG Problem

The ECD model assumes that the observed potentials are generated by a few current dipoles. The inverse EEG problem is to determine the position, orientation, and magnitude of these dipoles from the observed potentials.

From (6.4), it follows that

$$\mathcal{D}_{\Omega}(u|_{\partial\Omega}) = \sum_{s=1}^{m} \frac{\mathbf{q}_s \cdot (x - z_s)}{4\pi|x - z_s|^3} \quad \text{for } x \in \mathbb{R}^3 \setminus \overline{\Omega} \,.$$

The problem of localizing the dipoles $\mathbf{q}_s \delta_{z_s}$ can be formulated in terms of finding a least-squares fit of current dipoles to $\mathcal{D}_{\Omega}(u|_{\partial\Omega})$ outside Ω, which depends nonlinearly on the dipole positions.

6.3 The Spherical Model in MEG

The spherical model in MEG is routinely used in most clinical and research applications to MEG/EEG source localization.

Sarvas [112] has solved the inverse MEG problem for the spherical model completely in a very elegant way. Actually, for a conductive sphere of radius R with constant conductivity γ and a dipole of moment $\mathbf{q}$ located at a point z, the Geselowitz formula (6.7) reads

$$\mathbf{B}(x) = \frac{\mu}{4\pi}\mathbf{q} \times \frac{x-z}{|x-z|^3} - \frac{\mu\gamma}{4\pi R}\int_{\partial\Omega} u(y) \times \frac{y \times x}{|x-y|^3}\mathrm{d}\sigma(y) \,, \qquad (6.8)$$

for every x with $|x| > R$. What Sarvas observed is that the radial component of $\mathbf{B}$ is independent of the electric potential u and therefore it is known. In fact,

$$x \cdot \mathbf{B}(x) = \frac{\mu}{4\pi} \times \frac{x \cdot (z \times \mathbf{q})}{|x-z|^3} \quad \text{for } |x| > R \,.$$

Since $\mathbf{B}$ is irrotational outside Ω there exists a magnetic potential U, which decays as $|x|^{-2}$ at infinity, such that

$$\mathbf{B}(x) = \mu\nabla U(x) \quad \text{for } |x| > R \,. \qquad (6.9)$$

The crucial point now is that this potential U can be obtained from the known radial component of $\mathbf{B}$ alone. Indeed, an integration along the ray given by $x + t\hat{x}$, for $\hat{x} = x/R$, and $t \in [0, +\infty[$ yields

$$U(x) = -\int_0^{+\infty} \partial_t U(x + t\hat{x})\mathrm{d}t$$

$$= -\int_0^{+\infty} \hat{x} \cdot \nabla U(x + t\hat{x})\mathrm{d}t$$

$$= -\frac{1}{\mu}\int_0^{+\infty} \hat{x} \cdot \mathbf{B}(x + t\hat{x})\mathrm{d}t$$

$$= -\frac{1}{4\pi}\hat{x} \cdot (z \times \mathbf{q})\int_0^{+\infty} \frac{\mathrm{d}t}{|x + t\hat{x} - z|^3}$$

$$= -\frac{1}{4\pi}\hat{x} \cdot (z \times \mathbf{q})\frac{|x|}{F(x, z)}$$

$$= \frac{1}{4\pi}\frac{x \cdot (\mathbf{q} \times z)}{F(x, z)} \,,$$

where

$$F(x, z) = |x - z|\left[|x||x - z| + x \cdot (x - z)\right] \,.$$

Therefore, it follows from (6.9) that

$$\mathbf{B}(x) = \frac{\mu}{4\pi} \nabla \left(\frac{x \cdot (\mathbf{q} \times z)}{F(x,z)} \right) \quad \text{for } |x| > R \,. \tag{6.10}$$

Note that in this calculation for U, and therefore for $\mathbf{B}$ as well, the radius R of the sphere is not present. A more careful observation though reveals that this is a consequence of the fact that by using the radial component of $\mathbf{B}$ alone, the surface integral in equation (6.8), which provides the contribution of the conductive medium, disappears. Hence, the effect of the interface between the conducting and the non-conducting medium is eliminated. In other words, the symmetry is so high that the $\mathbf{B}$ field does not see the sphere. The conductive medium is transparent to the $\mathbf{B}$ field. We know though that this is not true for less symmetric domains such as an ellipsoid where this interface appears in the corresponding expressions.

It is an immediate consequence of (6.10) that if the direction of the moment becomes radial then $\mathbf{B}$ is zero in every point x outside the sphere. Radially oriented dipoles do not produce any external magnetic field outside a spherically symmetric volume conductor. Such dipole sources are called silent. Importantly, this is not the case for EEG, which is sensitive to radial sources, constituting one of the major differences between MEG and EEG.

The most classical MEG reconstruction algorithm is based on finding a least-squares fit of current dipoles to the observed $\mathbf{B}$-data.

Bibliography and Discussion

The least-squares method works reasonably well in EEG/MEG for source models with one or perhaps two dipoles but rapidly become more expensive to compute and less reliable as the number of dipoles increases. See [30, 125].

An alternative approach to ECD model is a diffuse current distribution, which can be discretized in terms of a large number of homogeneously distributed current dipoles. Models of this type have the advantage that the source structure need not be defined in advance. However, the number of model parameters is generally much larger than the number of measurement points, and so a solution has to be selected among an infinite number of possible solutions. To choose a meaningful solution from all possible solutions, we need to invoke a strong regularization scheme.

Realistic volume-conductor modeling of the head for accurate solution of the forward problem is needed. The derivation of the head model for the inverse source imaging can be done by integrating EEG/MEG with MRI. Surface boundaries for brain, skull, and scalp can be extracted from MR images.

In [122, 123], the finite element method is used for the forward problem. It allows realistic representation of the complicated head volume conductor.

In the case of a ECD model for the brain activity, the singularity of the potential at the source position is treated with the so-called subtraction dipole model; the model divides the total potential into the analytically known singularity potential and the singularity-free correction potential, which can then be approximated numerically with a finite element approach. However, most of the head models consider typical values for the conductivity of the brain, skull, and skin. These values are measured in vitro, where conductivity can be significantly altered compared to in vivo values. EIT may be used to estimate the conductivity profile. By injecting a small current between pairs of EEG electrodes and measuring the resulting potentials at all electrodes, EIT techniques can be used to reconstruct the conductivity values given a model for the head geometry.

We recommend [68] for a thorough review on MEG theory and instrumentation. We also refer to [23, 99] for excellent reviews on the underlying models currently used in MEG/EEG source estimation and on the imaging approaches to the inverse problem. The non-uniqueness question in the inverse MEG problem is discussed in [57, 58, 45, 46].

Part III

Anomaly Detection Algorithms

7

Small Volume Expansions

As shown in Sect. 5.1, in its most general form EIT is severely ill-posed and nonlinear. These are the main obstacles to find non-iterative reconstruction algorithms. If, however, in advance we have additional structural information about the conductivity profile, then we may be able to determine specific features about the conductivity distribution with a satisfactory resolution. One such type of knowledge could be that the body consists of a smooth background containing a number of unknown small anomalies with a significantly different conductivity. These anomalies might represent potential tumors.

Over the last 10 years or so, a considerable amount of interesting work has been dedicated to the imaging of such low volume fraction anomalies. The method of asymptotic expansions provides a useful framework to accurately and efficiently reconstruct the location and geometric features of the anomalies in a stable way, even for moderately noisy data. Using the method of matched asymptotic expansions we formally derive the first-order perturbations due to the presence of the anomalies. These perturbations are of dipole-type. A rigorous proof of these expansions is based on layer potential techniques. The concept of polarization tensor (PT) is the basic building block for the asymptotic expansion of the boundary perturbations. It is then important from an imaging point of view to precisely characterize the PT and derive some of its properties, such as symmetry, positivity, and optimal bounds on its elements, for developing efficient algorithms to reconstruct conductivity anomalies of small volume.

We then provide the leading-order term in this asymptotic formula of the solution to the Helmholtz equation in the presence of small electromagnetic (or acoustical) anomalies.

We extend the method of small volume expansions to isotropic elasticity. We derive the leading order term in the displacement perturbations due the presence of a small elastic anomaly in a homogeneous elastic body. The concept of PT is extended to elasticity defining the elastic moment tensor (EM). We provide some important properties of the EMT such as symmetry and positive-definiteness. We give an explicit formula for EMT associated with anomalies of elliptic shape. Our derivations can again be made rigorous based on layer potential techniques.

We also consider the elasticity problem in a quasi-incompressible body. We show that the elasticity system can be replaced with a nonhomogeneous modified Stokes system. We then (formally) establish an asymptotic development of the displacement field perturbations that are due to the presence of a small volume elastic anomaly. To construct this asymptotic expansion, we introduce the concept of viscous moment tensor (VMT). Connections between on one side the VMT and on the other side the EMT as well as the PT are given.

It is worth emphasizing that all the problems considered in this chapter are singularly perturbed problems. As it will be shown later, derivatives of the solution to the perturbed problem are not, inside the anomaly, close to those of the background solution. Consequently, a uniform expansion of the solution to the perturbed problem can not be constructed in the whole background domain. An example of a regularly perturbed problem is the Born approximation. See (5.5).

7.1 Conductivity Problem

In this section we derive an asymptotic expansion of the voltage potentials in the presence of a diametrically small anomaly with conductivity different from the background conductivity.

Consider the solution u of

$$
\begin{cases}
\nabla \cdot \left(\chi(\Omega \setminus \overline{D}) + k\chi(D) \right) \nabla u = 0 & \text{in } \Omega, \\
\dfrac{\partial u}{\partial \nu}\bigg|_{\partial \Omega} = g.
\end{cases}
\tag{7.1}
$$

The following asymptotic expansion expresses the fact that the conductivity anomaly can be modeled by a dipole.

Theorem 7.1.1 (Voltage Boundary Perturbations) *Suppose that* $D = \delta B + z$, *and let* u *be the solution of* (7.1), *where* $0 < k \neq 1 < +\infty$. *Denote* $\lambda := (k+1)/(2(k-1))$. *The following pointwise asymptotic expansion on* $\partial \Omega$ *holds for* $d = 2, 3$:

$$
u(x) = U(x) - \delta^d \nabla U(z) M(\lambda, B) \partial_z N(x, z) + O(\delta^{d+1}),
\tag{7.2}
$$

where the remainder $O(\delta^{d+1})$ *is dominated by* $C\delta^{d+1}\|g\|_{L^2(\partial\Omega)}$ *for some* C *independent of* $x \in \partial\Omega$. *Here* U *is the background solution,* $N(x, z)$ *is the Neumann function, that is, the solution to* (3.22), $M(\lambda, B) = (m_{pq})_{p,q=1}^d$ *is the polarization tensor (PT) given by*

$$m_{pq} = \int_{\partial B} (\lambda I - \mathcal{K}_B^*)^{-1}(\nu_p)\,\xi_q\,d\sigma(\xi)\,, \tag{7.3}$$

where $\nu = (\nu_1, \ldots, \nu_d), \xi = (\xi_1, \ldots, \xi_d)$.

7.1.1 Formal Derivations

To reveal the nature of the perturbations in the solution u to (7.1) that are due to the presence of the anomaly D, we introduce the local variables $\xi = (y-z)/\delta$ for $y \in \Omega$, and set $\hat{u}(\xi) = u(z+\delta\xi)$. We expect that $u(y)$ will differ appreciably from $U(y)$ for y near z, but it will differ little from $U(y)$ for y far from z. Therefore, using the method of matched asymptotic expansions, we represent the field u by two different expansions, an inner expansion for y near z, and an outer expansion for y far from z. The outer expansion must begin with U, so we write:

$$u(y) = U(y) + \delta^{\tau_1} U_1(y) + \delta^{\tau_2} U_2(y) + \ldots, \quad \text{for } |y - z| \gg O(\delta)\,,$$

where $0 < \tau_1 < \tau_2 < \ldots, U_1, U_2, \ldots$, are to be found.

We write the inner expansion as

$$\hat{u}(\xi) = u(z + \delta\xi) = \hat{u}_0(\xi) + \delta\hat{u}_1(\xi) + \delta^2\hat{u}_2(\xi) + \ldots, \quad \text{for } |\xi| = O(1)\,,$$

where $\hat{u}_0, \hat{u}_1, \ldots$, are to be found. We suppose that the functions $\hat{u}_j, j = 0, 1, \ldots$, are defined not just in the domain obtained by stretching Ω, but everywhere in $\mathbb{R}^d$.

Evidently, the functions $\hat{u}_i$ are not defined uniquely, and the question of how to choose them now arises. Thus, there is an arbitrariness in the choice of the coefficients of both the outer and the inner expansions. In order to determine the functions $U_i(y)$ and $\hat{u}_i(\xi)$, we have to equate the inner and the outer expansions in some overlap domain within which the stretched variable ξ is large and $y - z$ is small. In this domain the matching conditions are:

$$U(y) + \delta^{\tau_1} U_1(y) + \delta^{\tau_2} U_2(y) + \ldots \sim \hat{u}_0(\xi) + \delta\hat{u}_1(\xi) + \delta^2\hat{u}_2(\xi) + \ldots\,.$$

If we substitute the inner expansion into the transmission problem (7.1) and formally equate coefficients of δ^{-2}, δ^{-1} we get $\hat{u}_0(\xi) = U(z)$, and

$$\hat{u}_1(\xi) = \hat{v}_1(\frac{x-z}{\delta}) \cdot \nabla U(z)\,,$$

where

$$\begin{cases} \Delta\hat{v}_1 = 0 & \text{in } \mathbb{R}^d \setminus \overline{B}\,, \\ \Delta\hat{v}_1 = 0 & \text{in } B\,, \\ \hat{v}_1|_- - \hat{v}_1|_+ = 0 & \text{on } \partial B\,, \\ k\dfrac{\partial\hat{v}_1}{\partial\nu}|_- - \dfrac{\partial\hat{v}_1}{\partial\nu}|_+ = 0 & \text{on } \partial B\,, \\ \hat{v}_1(\xi) - \xi \to 0 & \text{as } |\xi| \to +\infty\,. \end{cases} \tag{7.4}$$

Therefore, we arrive at the following inner asymptotic formula:

$$u(x) \approx U(z) + \delta \hat{v}_1\left(\frac{x-z}{\delta}\right) \cdot \nabla U(z) \quad \text{for } x \text{ near } z . \tag{7.5}$$

Clearly, $\sup_{D} \|\nabla u(x) - \nabla U(x)\|$ does not approach zero as α goes to zero, and therefore, the problem is singulary perturbed.

Note also that

$$\hat{v}_1(\xi) = \xi + \mathcal{S}_B(\lambda I - \mathcal{K}_B^*)^{-1}(\nu), \quad \xi \in \mathbb{R}^d .$$

We now derive the outer expansion. From (3.38) we have

$$u(x) = H(x) + (k-1) \int_D \nabla_y \Gamma(x-y) \cdot \nabla u(y) \, dy .$$

Since

$$H(x) = -\mathcal{S}_\Omega g + \mathcal{D}_\Omega(u|_{\partial\Omega}) = U(x) + \mathcal{D}_\Omega((u-U)|_{\partial\Omega}), \quad x \in \Omega ,$$

then, by the jump relation (3.17), it follows that

$$\left(\frac{1}{2} - \mathcal{K}_\Omega\right)((u-U)|_{\partial\Omega}) = (k-1) \int_D \nabla_y \Gamma(x-y) \cdot \nabla u(y) \, dy .$$

Applying Lemma 3.1.11, we obtain that

$$(u - U)(x) = (1-k) \int_D \nabla_y N(x-y) \cdot \nabla u(y) \, dy$$

$$\approx (1-k) \nabla_y N(x,z) \cdot \int_D \nabla u(y) \, dy ,$$

for $x \in \partial\Omega$. By using the inner expansion, we arrive at the outer expansion:

$$u(x) \approx U(x) + \delta^d (1-k) \nabla_y N(x,z)\left(\int_B \nabla \hat{v}_1(\xi) \, d\xi\right) \cdot \nabla U(z), \quad x \in \partial\Omega .$$

Next, compute

$$\int_B \nabla \hat{v}_1(\xi) \, d\xi = \int_B (I + \nabla \mathcal{S}_B(\lambda I - \mathcal{K}_B^*)^{-1}(\nu)) \, d\xi$$

$$= |B|I + \int_{\partial B} \left(-\frac{I}{2} + \mathcal{K}_B^*\right)(\lambda I - \mathcal{K}_B^*)^{-1}(\nu)\xi \, d\sigma(\xi)$$

$$= \frac{1}{k-1} \int_{\partial B} (\lambda I - \mathcal{K}_B^*)^{-1}(\nu) \, \xi \, d\sigma(\xi) ,$$

and therefore,

$$u(x) \approx U(x) - \delta^d \nabla_y N(x,z) M(\lambda, B) \cdot \nabla U(z), \quad x \in \partial\Omega , \tag{7.6}$$

where $M(k,B)$ is the polarization tensor associated with B and the conductivity $k = (2\lambda + 1)/(2\lambda - 1)$ defined by (7.3).

7.1.2 Polarization Tensor

The polarization tensor M can be explicitly computed for disks and ellipses in the plane and balls and ellipsoids in three-dimensional space.

Let $|\lambda| > 1/2$ and let $k = (2\lambda + 1)/(2\lambda - 1)$. If B is an ellipse whose semi-axes are on the x_1- and x_2-axes and of length a and b, respectively, then its polarization tensor M takes the form

$$M(\lambda, B) = (k - 1)|B| \begin{pmatrix} \dfrac{a+b}{a+kb} & 0 \\ 0 & \dfrac{a+b}{b+ka} \end{pmatrix} , \qquad (7.7)$$

where $|B|$ denotes the volume of B.

For an arbitrary ellipse whose semi-axes are not aligned with the coordinate axes, one can use the identity

$$M(\lambda, \mathcal{R}B) = \mathcal{R}M(\lambda, B)\mathcal{R}^T \quad \text{for any unitary transformation } \mathcal{R},$$

to compute its polarization tensor.

In the three-dimensional case, a domain for which analogous analytical expressions for the elements of its polarization tensor M are available is the ellipsoid. If the coordinate axes are chosen to coincide with the principal axes of the ellipsoid B whose equation then becomes

$$\frac{x_1^2}{a^2} + \frac{x_2^2}{b^2} + \frac{x_3^2}{c^2} = 1, \quad 0 < c \le b \le a ,$$

then M takes the form

$$M(\lambda, B) = (k-1)|B| \begin{pmatrix} \dfrac{1}{(1-A)+kA} & 0 & 0 \\ 0 & \dfrac{1}{(1-B)+kB} & 0 \\ 0 & 0 & \dfrac{1}{(1-C)+kC} \end{pmatrix} , \quad (7.8)$$

where the constants $A, B,$ and C are defined by

$$A = \frac{bc}{a^2} \int_1^{+\infty} \frac{1}{t^2 \sqrt{t^2 - 1 + (\frac{b}{a})^2} \sqrt{t^2 - 1 + (\frac{c}{a})^2}} \, dt ,$$

$$B = \frac{bc}{a^2} \int_1^{+\infty} \frac{1}{(t^2 - 1 + (\frac{b}{a})^2)^{\frac{3}{2}} \sqrt{t^2 - 1 + (\frac{c}{a})^2}} \, dt ,$$

$$C = \frac{bc}{a^2} \int_1^{+\infty} \frac{1}{\sqrt{t^2 - 1 + (\frac{b}{a})^2} (t^2 - 1 + (\frac{c}{a})^2)^{\frac{3}{2}}} \, dt .$$

In the special case, $a = b = c$, the ellipsoid B becomes a sphere and $A = B = C = 1/3$. Hence the polarization tensor associated with the sphere B is given by

$$M(\lambda, B) = (k-1)|B| \begin{pmatrix} \dfrac{3}{2+k} & 0 & 0 \\ 0 & \dfrac{3}{2+k} & 0 \\ 0 & 0 & \dfrac{3}{2+k} \end{pmatrix}.$$

We now list important properties of the PT.

Theorem 7.1.2 (Properties of the Polarization Tensor) *For $|\lambda| > 1/2$, let $M(\lambda, B) = (m_{pq})_{p,q=1}^{d}$ be the PT associated with the bounded domain B in $\mathbb{R}^d$ and the conductivity $k = (2\lambda + 1)/(2\lambda - 1)$. Then*

(i) *M is symmetric.*
(ii) *If $k > 1$, then M is positive definite, and it is negative definite if $0 < k < 1$.*
(iii) *The following optimal bounds for the PT*

$$\begin{cases} \dfrac{1}{k-1}\, \mathrm{trace}(M) \le (d - 1 + \dfrac{1}{k})|B|\,, \\ (k-1)\, \mathrm{trace}(M^{-1}) \le \dfrac{d - 1 + k}{|B|}\,, \end{cases} \tag{7.9}$$

hold, where trace *denotes the trace of a matrix.*

Note that by making use of bounds (7.9), an accurate size estimation of B can be immediately obtained.

It is also worth mentioning that in the literature on effective medium theory, the bounds (7.9) are known as the Hashin-Shtrikman bounds. The concept of polarization tensors appear in deriving asymptotic expansions of electrical effective properties of composite dilute media. Polarization tensors involve microstructural information beyond that contained in the volume fractions (material contrast, inclusion shape and orientation). See [16].

7.2 Helmholtz Equation

Suppose that an electromagnetic medium occupies a bounded domain Ω in $\mathbb{R}^d$, with a connected C^2-boundary $\partial\Omega$. Suppose that Ω contains a small anomaly of the form $D = \delta B + z$, where $z \in \Omega$ and B is a C^2-bounded domain in $\mathbb{R}^d$ containing the origin.

Let μ_0 and ε_0 denote the permeability and the permittivity of the background medium Ω, and assume that $\mu_0 > 0$ and $\varepsilon_0 > 0$ are positive constants.

Let $\mu_\star > 0$ and $\varepsilon_\star > 0$ denote the permeability and the permittivity of the anomaly D, which are also assumed to be positive constants. Introduce the piecewise-constant magnetic permeability

$$\mu_\delta(x) = \begin{cases} \mu_0 , & x \in \Omega \setminus \overline{D} , \\ \mu_\star , & x \in D . \end{cases}$$

The piecewise constant electric permittivity, $\varepsilon_\delta(x)$, is defined analogously.

Let the electric field u denote the solution to the Helmholtz equation

$$\nabla \cdot (\frac{1}{\mu_\delta} \nabla u) + \omega^2 \varepsilon_\delta u = 0 \quad \text{in } \Omega , \tag{7.10}$$

with the boundary condition $u = f \in W_{\frac{1}{2}}^2(\partial\Omega)$, where $\omega > 0$ is a given frequency.

Note that the use of the formal equivalence between electromagnetics and acoustics, by term-to-term replacing permittivity and permeability by compressibility and volume density of mass, and replacing the electric field by the acoustic pressure, opens up the investigation below to ultrasound imaging of small anomalies as well.

Problem (7.10) can be written as

$$\begin{cases} (\Delta + \omega^2 \varepsilon_0 \mu_0)u = 0 & \text{in } \Omega \setminus \overline{D} , \\ (\Delta + \omega^2 \varepsilon_\star \mu_\star)u = 0 & \text{in } D , \\ \dfrac{1}{\mu_\star} \dfrac{\partial u}{\partial \nu}\Big|_- - \dfrac{1}{\mu_0} \dfrac{\partial u}{\partial \nu}\Big|_+ = 0 & \text{on } \partial D , \\ u\big|_- - u\big|_+ = 0 & \text{on } \partial D , \\ u = f & \text{on } \partial\Omega . \end{cases}$$

Assume that

$$\omega^2 \varepsilon_0 \mu_0 \text{ is not an eigenvalue for the operator } -\Delta \text{ in } L^2(\Omega)$$

$$\text{with homogeneous Dirichlet boundary conditions,} \tag{7.11}$$

we can prove existence and uniqueness of a solution to (7.10) at least for δ small enough.

With the notation of Sect. 3.2, the following asymptotic formula holds.

Theorem 7.2.1 (Boundary Perturbations) *Suppose that (7.11) holds. Let u be the solution of (7.10) and let the function U be the background solution as before. For any $x \in \partial\Omega$,*

$$\frac{\partial u}{\partial \nu}(x) = \frac{\partial U}{\partial \nu}(x) + \delta^d \Bigg(\nabla U(z) M(\lambda, B) \frac{\partial \nabla_z G_{k_0}(x, z)}{\partial \nu_x}$$

$$+ \omega^2 \mu_0 (\varepsilon_\star - \varepsilon_0) |B| U(z) \frac{\partial G_{k_0}(x, z)}{\partial \nu_x} \Bigg) + O(\delta^{d+1}) , \tag{7.12}$$

where $M(\lambda, B)$ is the polarization tensor defined in (7.3) with λ given by

$$\lambda := \frac{(\mu_0/\mu_\star) + 1}{2((\mu_0/\mu_\star) - 1)} . \tag{7.13}$$

7.2.1 Formal Derivations

From the Lippman-Schwinger integral representation formula

$$u(x) = U(x) + (\frac{\mu_0}{\mu_\star} - 1) \int_D \nabla u(y) \cdot \nabla G_{k_0}(x, y) \, dy$$
$$+ k_0^2(\frac{\varepsilon_\star}{\varepsilon_0} - 1) \int_D u(y) G_{k_0}(x, y) \, dy, \quad x \in \Omega ,$$

it follows that for any $x \in \partial\Omega$,

$$\frac{\partial u}{\partial \nu}(x) = \frac{\partial U}{\partial \nu}(x) + (\frac{\mu_0}{\mu_\star} - 1) \int_D \nabla u(y) \cdot \frac{\partial \nabla_y G_{k_0}(x, y)}{\partial \nu_x} \, dy$$
$$+ k_0^2(\frac{\varepsilon_\star}{\varepsilon_0} - 1) \int_D u(y) \frac{\partial G_{k_0}(x, y)}{\partial \nu_x} \, dy .$$

Using a Taylor expansion of $G_{k_0}(x, y)$ for $y \in D$, we readily see that for any $x \in \partial\Omega$,

$$\frac{\partial u}{\partial \nu}(x) \approx \frac{\partial U}{\partial \nu}(x) + (\frac{\mu_0}{\mu_\star} - 1)\frac{\partial \nabla_z G_{k_0}(x, z)}{\partial \nu_x} \cdot (\int_D \nabla u(y) \, dy)$$
$$+ k_0^2(\frac{\varepsilon_\star}{\varepsilon_0} - 1)\frac{\partial G_{k_0}(x, z)}{\partial \nu_x}(\int_D u(y) \, dy) . \tag{7.14}$$

Following the same lines as in the derivation of the asymptotic expansion of the voltage potentials in Sect. 7.1, one can easily check that $u(y) \approx U(z)$, for $y \in D$, and

$$\int_D \nabla u(y) \, dy \approx \delta^d \left(\int_B \nabla \hat{v}_1(\xi) \, d\xi \right) \cdot \nabla U(z) ,$$

where $\hat{v}_1$ is defined by (7.4) with $k = \mu_0/\mu_\star$. Inserting these two approximations into (7.14) leads to (7.12).

7.3 Static Elasticity

Suppose that the elastic body occupies a bounded C^2-domain Ω in $\mathbb{R}^d$, with a connected boundary $\partial\Omega$. Let the constants (λ, μ) denote the background Lamé coefficients, that are the elastic parameters in the absence of any anomalies. Suppose that the elastic anomaly D in Ω is given by $D = \delta B + z$, where B is a bounded $\mathcal{C}^2$-domain in $\mathbb{R}^d$. Suppose that D has the pair of Lamé constants $(\tilde{\lambda}, \tilde{\mu})$ satisfying (3.84) and (3.85).

The purpose of this section is to find an asymptotic expansion for the displacement field in terms of the reference Lamé constants, the location, and the shape of the anomaly D. This expansion describes the perturbation of the solution caused by the presence of D.

Consider the transmission problem

$$\begin{cases} \displaystyle\sum_{j,k,l=1}^{d} \frac{\partial}{\partial x_j}\left(C_{ijkl}\frac{\partial u_k}{\partial x_l}\right) = 0 \quad \text{in } \Omega, \quad i = 1,\dots,d\,, \\ \displaystyle\frac{\partial \mathbf{u}}{\partial \nu}\bigg|_{\partial\Omega} = \mathbf{g}\,, \end{cases} \tag{7.15}$$

where the elasticity tensor $C = (C_{ijkl})$ is given by

$$C_{ijkl} := \left(\lambda\,\chi(\Omega\setminus D) + \tilde{\lambda}\,\chi(D)\right)\delta_{ij}\delta_{kl}$$
$$+ \left(\mu\,\chi(\Omega\setminus D) + \tilde{\mu}\,\chi(D)\right)(\delta_{ik}\delta_{jl} + \delta_{il}\delta_{jk})\,,$$

and u_k for $k = 1,\dots,d$, denote the components of the displacement field $\mathbf{u}$.

In order to ensure existence and uniqueness of a solution to (7.15), we assume that $\mathbf{g} \in L^2_{\Psi}(\partial\Omega)$.

With the notation of Sect. 3.3, the following asymptotic formula holds.

Theorem 7.3.1 (Displacement Boundary Perturbations) *Let* $\mathbf{u}$ *be the solution of (7.15) and* $\mathbf{U}$ *the background solution. The following pointwise asymptotic expansion on* $\partial\Omega$ *holds:*

$$\mathbf{u}(x) = \mathbf{U}(x) - \delta^d \partial\mathbf{U}(z)\partial_z\mathbf{N}(x,z)M + O(\delta^{d+1})\,, \quad x \in \partial\Omega\,, \tag{7.16}$$

where $M = (m_{pq}^{ij})_{i,j,p,q=1,\dots,d}$ *is the elastic moment tensor (EMT) given by*

$$m_{pq}^{ij} = \int_{\partial B} \xi_p \mathbf{e}_q \cdot \mathbf{g}_i^j(\xi)\,d\sigma(\xi)\,. \tag{7.17}$$

Here $(\mathbf{e}_1,\dots,\mathbf{e}_d)$ *is an orthonormal basis of* $\mathbb{R}^d$ *and* $(\mathbf{f}_i^j, \mathbf{g}_i^j)$ *is the solution to*

$$\begin{cases} \tilde{\mathcal{S}}_B\mathbf{f}_i^j\big|_- - \mathcal{S}_B\mathbf{g}_i^j\big|_+ = \xi_i\mathbf{e}_j\big|_{\partial B}\,, \\ \dfrac{\partial}{\partial\tilde{\nu}}\tilde{\mathcal{S}}_B\mathbf{f}_i^j\bigg|_- - \dfrac{\partial}{\partial\nu}\mathcal{S}_B\mathbf{g}_i^j\bigg|_+ = \dfrac{\partial(\xi_i\mathbf{e}_j)}{\partial\nu}\big|_{\partial B}\,. \end{cases} \tag{7.18}$$

We note the analogy of the EMT with the PT. The expansion (7.16) can be rewritten as follows: For $x \in \partial\Omega$,

$$u_i(x) = U_i(x) - \delta^d \sum_{j,p,q=1}^{d} (\partial_p U_j)(z)\,\partial_{z_q} N_{ij}(x,z)\,m_{pq}^{ij}\,, \quad i = 1,\dots,d\,.$$

7.3.1 Formal Derivations

Using again the method of matched asymptotic expansions, we give a formal derivation of the leading-order term in the asymptotic expansion of the displacement field $\mathbf{u}$ as $\delta \to 0$. The outer expansion reads:

$$\mathbf{u}(y) = \mathbf{U}(y) + \delta^{\tau_1}\mathbf{U}_1(y) + \delta^{\tau_2}\mathbf{U}_2(y) + \ldots, \quad \text{for } |y - z| \gg O(\delta),$$

where $0 < \tau_1 < \tau_2 < \ldots$, $\mathbf{U}_1, \mathbf{U}_2, \ldots$, are to be found.

The inner expansion is written as

$$\hat{\mathbf{u}}(\xi) = \mathbf{u}(z + \delta\xi) = \hat{\mathbf{u}}_0(\xi) + \delta\hat{\mathbf{u}}_1(\xi) + \delta^2\hat{\mathbf{u}}_2(\xi) + \ldots, \quad \text{for } |\xi| = O(1),$$

where $\hat{\mathbf{u}}_0, \hat{\mathbf{u}}_1, \ldots$, are to be found.

In some overlap domain the matching conditions are:

$$\mathbf{U}(y) + \delta^{\tau_1}\mathbf{U}_1(y) + \delta^{\tau_2}\mathbf{U}_2(y) + \ldots \sim \hat{\mathbf{u}}_0(\xi) + \delta\hat{\mathbf{u}}_1(\xi) + \delta^2\hat{\mathbf{u}}_2(\xi) + \ldots.$$

If we substitute the inner expansion into the transmission problem (7.15) and formally equate coefficients of δ^{-2} and δ^{-1}, we get:

$$\hat{\mathbf{u}}_0(\xi) = \mathbf{U}(z), \quad \text{and} \quad \hat{\mathbf{u}}_1(\xi) = \sum (\partial_p U_j)(z)\hat{\mathbf{v}}_{1ij}(\xi),$$

where $\hat{\mathbf{v}}_{1ij}$ is the solution to

$$\begin{cases} \mathcal{L}_{\lambda,\mu}\hat{\mathbf{v}}_{1ij} = 0 & \text{in } \mathbb{R}^d \setminus \overline{B}, \\ \mathcal{L}_{\tilde{\lambda},\tilde{\mu}}\hat{\mathbf{v}}_{1ij} = 0 & \text{in } B, \\ \hat{\mathbf{v}}_{1ij}|_- - \hat{\mathbf{v}}_{1ij}|_+ = 0 & \text{on } \partial B, \\ \dfrac{\partial\hat{\mathbf{v}}_{1ij}}{\partial\tilde{\nu}}\bigg|_- - \dfrac{\partial\hat{\mathbf{v}}_{1ij}}{\partial\nu}\bigg|_+ = 0 & \text{on } \partial B, \\ \hat{\mathbf{v}}_{1ij}(\xi) - \xi_i\mathbf{e}_j \to 0 & \text{as } |\xi| \to +\infty. \end{cases} \qquad (7.19)$$

Therefore, we arrive at the following inner asymptotic formula:

$$\mathbf{u}(x) \approx \mathbf{U}(z) + \delta\sum_{i,j,p}\hat{\mathbf{v}}_{1ij}\left(\frac{x - z}{\delta}\right)(\partial_p U_j)(z) \quad \text{for } x \text{ near } z. \qquad (7.20)$$

Note that $\hat{\mathbf{v}}_{1ij}$ admits the following representation

$$\hat{\mathbf{v}}_{1ij}(\xi) = \begin{cases} \xi_i\mathbf{e}_j + \mathcal{S}_B\mathbf{g}_i^j(\xi) & \text{in } \mathbb{R}^d \setminus \overline{B}, \\ \tilde{\mathcal{S}}_B\mathbf{f}_i^j(\xi) & \text{in } B, \end{cases} \qquad (7.21)$$

where $(\mathbf{f}_i^j, \mathbf{g}_i^j)$ is the unique solution to (7.18).

We now derive the outer expansion. From (3.93),

$$\mathbf{u}(x) = \mathbf{H}(x) + \mathcal{S}_D\psi(x), \quad x \in \Omega \setminus \overline{D},$$

where $\psi \in L^2_{\bar{\psi}}(\partial D)$ and $\mathbf{H}(x) = \mathcal{D}_\Omega(\mathbf{u}|_{\partial\Omega})(x) - \mathcal{S}_\Omega(\mathbf{g})(x)$, which yields

$$(\frac{I}{2} - \mathcal{K}_\Omega)((\mathbf{u} - \mathbf{U})|_{\partial\Omega}) = \mathcal{S}_D\psi \quad \text{on } \partial\Omega .$$

By using the jump relation (3.78),

$$\psi = \partial\mathcal{S}_D\psi/\partial\nu|_+ - \partial\mathcal{S}_D\psi/\partial\nu|_- . \tag{7.22}$$

Combining (7.22) together with the transmission conditions (3.95), and Green's identity

$$\int_{\partial D} \left(\mathbf{\Gamma}\frac{\partial\mathbf{H}}{\partial\nu} - \frac{\partial\mathbf{\Gamma}}{\partial\nu}\mathbf{H} \right) d\sigma = 0 ,$$

we get

$$\mathcal{S}_D\psi = \int_{\partial D} \left(\mathbf{\Gamma}\frac{\partial\tilde{\mathcal{S}}_D\varphi}{\partial\tilde{\nu}}|_- - \frac{\partial\mathbf{\Gamma}}{\partial\nu}\tilde{\mathcal{S}}_D\varphi \right) d\sigma \quad \text{on } \partial\Omega .$$

Thus,

$$\mathcal{S}_D\psi = (\tilde{\lambda} - \lambda)\int_D \nabla \cdot \mathbf{\Gamma}\nabla \cdot \mathbf{u} + \frac{(\tilde{\mu} - \mu)}{2}\int_D (\nabla\mathbf{\Gamma} + \nabla\mathbf{\Gamma}^T) \cdot (\nabla\mathbf{u} + \nabla\mathbf{u}^T) .$$

Inserting the inner expansion (7.20) into the above identity and using Lemma 3.3.11, we obtain after expanding

$$\mathbf{N}(x, y) \approx \mathbf{N}(x, z) + \nabla\mathbf{N}(x, z) \cdot (x - z) \quad \text{for } y \in \partial D ,$$

that for any $x \in \partial\Omega$,

$$(\mathbf{u} - \mathbf{U})(x) \approx -\delta^d\nabla\mathbf{N}(x, z)\left[(\tilde{\lambda} - \lambda)(\int_B \nabla \cdot (\xi_p\mathbf{e}_q) \nabla \cdot \hat{\mathbf{v}}_{1ij}(\xi)\, d\xi) + \frac{(\tilde{\mu} - \mu)}{2}\right.$$
$$\left. \times \left(\int_B (\nabla(\xi_p\mathbf{e}_q) + \nabla(\xi_p\mathbf{e}_q)^T) \cdot (\nabla\hat{\mathbf{v}}_{1ij}(\xi) + (\nabla\hat{\mathbf{v}}_{1ij}(\xi))^T)\, d\xi \right) \right] (\partial_p U_j)(z) .$$

Since $\xi_p\mathbf{e}_q$ is linear, integrating by parts gives

$$(\tilde{\lambda} - \lambda)(\int_B \nabla \cdot (\xi_p\mathbf{e}_q) \nabla \cdot \hat{\mathbf{v}}_{1ij}(\xi)\, d\xi)$$
$$+ \frac{(\tilde{\mu} - \mu)}{2}\left(\int_B (\nabla(\xi_p\mathbf{e}_q) + \nabla(\xi_p\mathbf{e}_q)^T) \cdot (\nabla\hat{\mathbf{v}}_{1ij}(\xi) + (\nabla\hat{\mathbf{v}}_{1ij}(\xi))^T)\, d\xi \right)$$
$$= \int_{\partial B} \hat{\mathbf{v}}_{1ij}(\xi) \cdot \left(\frac{\partial}{\partial\tilde{\nu}} - \frac{\partial}{\partial\nu} \right)(\xi_p\mathbf{e}_q)\, d\sigma(\xi) .$$

But, from (7.21) it follows again by integrating by parts that

$$\int_{\partial B} \hat{\mathbf{v}}_{1ij} \cdot \left(\frac{\partial}{\partial\tilde{\nu}} - \frac{\partial}{\partial\nu} \right)(\xi_p\mathbf{e}_q)\, d\sigma$$
$$= \int_{\partial B} \left(\frac{\partial}{\partial\tilde{\nu}}\tilde{\mathcal{S}}_B\mathbf{f}_i^j \Big|_- - \frac{\partial}{\partial\nu}(\xi_i\mathbf{e}_j + \mathcal{S}_B\mathbf{g}_i^j)\Big|_- \right)\xi_p\mathbf{e}_q\, d\sigma$$
$$= \int_{\partial B} \left(\frac{\partial}{\partial\nu}\mathcal{S}_B\mathbf{g}_i^j \Big|_+ - \frac{\partial}{\partial\nu}\mathcal{S}_B\mathbf{g}_i^j \Big|_- \right)\xi_p\mathbf{e}_q\, d\sigma$$
$$= m_{pq}^{ij} ,$$

as desired.

7.3.2 Elastic Moment Tensor

Let (m_{pq}^{ij}) be the EMT for the ellipse B whose semi-axes are on the x_1- and x_2-axes and of length a and b, respectively, and let $(\tilde{\lambda}, \tilde{\mu})$ and (λ, μ) be the Lamé parameters of B and the background, respectively.

Then we have

$$m_{11}^{11} = |B|(\lambda + 2\mu)\frac{(\tilde{\mu} - \mu)(\tilde{\lambda} - \lambda + \tilde{\mu} - \mu)[m^2 - 2(\tau - 1)m] + c}{(\tilde{\mu} - \mu)[3\mu + (1 - \tau)(\tilde{\lambda} + \tilde{\mu})]m^2 + (\mu + \tilde{\lambda} + \tilde{\mu})(\mu + \tau\tilde{\mu})} ,$$

$$m_{22}^{22} = |B|(\lambda + 2\mu)\frac{(\tilde{\mu} - \mu)(\tilde{\lambda} - \lambda + \tilde{\mu} - \mu)[m^2 + 2(\tau - 1)m] + c}{(\tilde{\mu} - \mu)[3\mu + (1 - \tau)(\tilde{\lambda} + \tilde{\mu})]m^2 + (\mu + \tilde{\lambda} + \tilde{\mu})(\mu + \tau\tilde{\mu})} ,$$

$$m_{22}^{11} = |B|\frac{(\lambda + 2\mu)[(\tilde{\mu} - \mu)(\tilde{\lambda} - \lambda + \tilde{\mu} - \mu)m^2 + (\tilde{\lambda} - \lambda)(\tilde{\mu} + \tau\mu) + (\tilde{\mu} - \mu)^2]}{(\tilde{\mu} - \mu)[3\mu + (1 - \tau)(\tilde{\lambda} + \tilde{\mu})]m^2 + (\mu + \tilde{\lambda} + \tilde{\mu})(\mu + \tau\tilde{\mu})} ,$$

$$m_{12}^{12} = |B|\frac{\mu(\tilde{\mu} - \mu)(\tau + 1)}{-(\tilde{\mu} - \mu)m^2 + \mu + \tau\tilde{\mu}} ,$$

where

$$c = (\tilde{\lambda} - \lambda + \tilde{\mu} - \mu)(\mu + \tau\tilde{\mu}) + (\tau - 1)(\tilde{\mu} - \mu)(\mu + \tilde{\lambda} + \tilde{\mu}) ,$$

$m = (a - b)/(a + b)$ and $\tau = (\lambda + 3\mu)/(\lambda + \mu)$. In particular, if $m = 0$, i.e., B is a disk, then

$$\begin{cases} m_{22}^{11} = |B|\frac{(\lambda + 2\mu)[(\tilde{\lambda} - \lambda)(\tilde{\mu} + \tau\mu) + (\tilde{\mu} - \mu)^2]}{(\mu + \tilde{\lambda} + \tilde{\mu})(\mu + \tau\tilde{\mu})} , \\ m_{12}^{12} = |B|\frac{\mu(\tilde{\mu} - \mu)(\tau + 1)}{\mu + \tau\tilde{\mu}} . \end{cases} \qquad (7.23)$$

We now provide some important properties of the EMT such as symmetry, positive-definiteness, and optimal bounds. Let us fix a notation first. In $\mathbb{R}^d$, $d = 2, 3$, let

$$\mathbf{I}_2 := \delta_{ij}\mathbf{e}_i \otimes \mathbf{e}_j ,$$

$$\mathbf{I}_4 := \frac{1}{2}(\delta_{ik}\delta_{jl} + \delta_{il}\delta_{jk})\mathbf{e}_i \otimes \mathbf{e}_j \otimes \mathbf{e}_k \otimes \mathbf{e}_l .$$

Here, $\mathbf{I}_2$ is the $d \times d$ identity matrix or 2-tensor while $\mathbf{I}_4$ is the identity 4-tensor. Set

$$\mathbf{\Lambda}_1 := \frac{1}{d}\mathbf{I}_2 \otimes \mathbf{I}_2, \quad \mathbf{\Lambda}_2 := \mathbf{I}_4 - \mathbf{\Lambda}_1 . \qquad (7.24)$$

Since for any $d \times d$ symmetric matrix A

$$\mathbf{I}_2 \otimes \mathbf{I}_2(A) = (A : \mathbf{I}_2)\,\mathbf{I}_2 = \text{trace}(A)\,\mathbf{I}_2 \quad \text{and} \quad \mathbf{I}_4(A) = A ,$$

one can immediately see that

$$\Lambda_1\Lambda_1 = \Lambda_1, \quad \Lambda_2\Lambda_2 = \Lambda_2, \quad \Lambda_1\Lambda_2 = 0 .$$

With this notation, the EMT of a disk is given by

$$M = 2|B|\frac{(\lambda + 2\mu)(\tilde{\lambda} + \tilde{\mu} - \lambda - \mu)}{\mu + \tilde{\lambda} + \tilde{\mu}}\Lambda_1 + 2|B|\frac{\mu(\tilde{\mu} - \mu)(\tau + 1)}{\mu + \tau\tilde{\mu}}\Lambda_2 . \quad (7.25)$$

The following holds.

Theorem 7.3.2 (Properties of the Elastic Moment Tensor) *Let M be the EMT associated with the domain B, and $(\tilde{\lambda}, \tilde{\mu})$ and (λ, μ) be the Lamé parameters of B and the background, respectively. Set $\kappa = \lambda + 2\mu/d, \tilde{\kappa} = \tilde{\lambda} + 2\tilde{\mu}/d$. Then,*

(i) *For $p, q, i, j = 1, \ldots, d$, the following holds:*

$$m_{pq}^{ij} = m_{qp}^{ij}, \quad m_{pq}^{ij} = m_{pq}^{ji}, \quad \text{and} \quad m_{pq}^{ij} = m_{ij}^{pq} . \quad (7.26)$$

(ii) *Suppose that (3.85) holds. If $\tilde{\mu} > \mu$ ($\tilde{\mu} < \mu$, resp.), then M is positive (negative, resp.) definite on the space M_d^S of $d \times d$ symmetric matrices.*

(iii) *Suppose for simplicity that $\tilde{\mu} > \mu$. We have*

$$\frac{1}{|B|}\text{Tr}(\Lambda_1 M\Lambda_1) \le d(\tilde{\kappa} - \kappa)\frac{d\kappa + 2(d-1)\tilde{\mu}}{d\tilde{\kappa} + 2(d-1)\tilde{\mu}} \quad (7.27)$$

$$\frac{1}{|B|}\text{Tr}(\Lambda_2 M\Lambda_2) \le 2(\tilde{\mu} - \mu)\left[\frac{d^2 + d - 2}{2}\right.$$
$$\left. - 2(\tilde{\mu} - \mu)\left(\frac{d-1}{2\tilde{\mu}} + \frac{d-1}{d\tilde{\kappa} + 2(d-1)\tilde{\mu}}\right)\right], \quad (7.28)$$

$$|B|\,\text{Tr}\left(\Lambda_1 M^{-1}\Lambda_1\right) \le \frac{1}{d(\tilde{\kappa} - \kappa)}\frac{d\tilde{\kappa} + 2(d-1)\mu}{d\kappa + 2(d-1)\mu}, \quad (7.29)$$

$$|B|\,\text{Tr}\left(\Lambda_2 M^{-1}\Lambda_2\right) \le \frac{1}{2(\tilde{\mu} - \mu)}\left[\frac{d^2 + d - 2}{2}\right.$$
$$\left. + 2(\tilde{\mu} - \mu)\left(\frac{d-1}{2\mu} + \frac{d-1}{d\kappa + 2(d-1)\mu}\right)\right], \quad (7.30)$$

where for $C = (C_{ij}^{pq})$, $\text{Tr}(C) := \sum_{i,j=1}^d C_{ij}^{ij}$.

Note that $\text{Tr}(\Lambda_1) = 1$ and $\text{Tr}(\Lambda_2) = (d(d+1) - 2)/2$. The symmetry property (7.26) implies that M is a symmetric linear transformation on the space M_d^S. The bounds (7.27)–(7.30) are called Hashin-Shtrikman bounds for the EMT.

7.4 Dynamic Elasticity

Let ρ and $\tilde{\rho}$ be two positive constants. Physically, ρ and $\tilde{\rho}$ denote the densities of the background and the anomaly, respectively. Consider the transmission problem

$$
\begin{cases}
\mathcal{L}_{\lambda,\mu}\mathbf{u} + \omega^2 \rho \mathbf{u} = 0 & \text{in } \Omega \setminus \overline{D} , \\
\mathcal{L}_{\tilde{\lambda},\tilde{\mu}}\mathbf{u} + \omega^2 \tilde{\rho}\mathbf{u} = 0 & \text{in } D , \\
\dfrac{\partial \mathbf{u}}{\partial \nu} = \mathbf{g} & \text{on } \partial\Omega , \\
\mathbf{u}\big|_+ - \mathbf{u}\big|_- = 0 & \text{on } \partial D , \\
\dfrac{\partial \mathbf{u}}{\partial \nu}\big|_+ - \dfrac{\partial \mathbf{u}}{\partial \tilde{\nu}}\big|_- = 0 & \text{on } \partial D .
\end{cases}
\tag{7.31}
$$

Suppose that

$$
\omega^2 \rho \text{ is not an eigenvalue for the operator } -\mathcal{L}_{\lambda,\mu} \text{ in } L^2(\Omega)
$$
$$
\text{with homogeneous Neumann boundary conditions,}
$$

we can prove existence and uniqueness of a solution to (7.31) for δ small enough.

Let $\mathbf{N}^\omega(x,y)$ be the Neumann function for $\mathcal{L}_{\lambda,\mu} + \omega^2 \rho$ in Ω corresponding to a Dirac mass at y. That is, $\mathbf{N}^\omega$ is the solution to

$$
\begin{cases}
\mathcal{L}_{\lambda,\mu}\mathbf{N}^\omega(x,y) + \omega^2 \rho\mathbf{N}^\omega(x,y) = -\delta_y(x)I_d & \text{in } \Omega , \\
\dfrac{\partial \mathbf{N}}{\partial \nu}\bigg|_{\partial\Omega} = 0 .
\end{cases}
$$

Following the same lines as in the derivation in the static case of the asymptotic expansion of the displacement field as $\delta \to$, we find that for any $x \in \partial\Omega$,

$$
\mathbf{u}(x) = \mathbf{U}(x) - \delta^d\left[\partial\mathbf{U}(z)\partial_z\mathbf{N}^\omega(x,z)M + \omega^2(\rho-\tilde{\rho})|B|\mathbf{N}^\omega(x,z)\mathbf{U}(z)\right] + O(\delta^{d+1}) ,
$$

where M is the EMT associated with B and the pairs of Lamé coefficients (λ,μ) and $(\tilde{\lambda},\tilde{\mu})$.

7.5 Modified Stokes System

In soft tissues, quasi-incompressibility leads to $\lambda \gg \mu$ and thus the compression waves propagate much faster than the shear waves. To remove λ from consideration, we replace the elasticity system in biological tissues with a sequence of nonhomogeneous modified Stokes systems. Then we derive the leading-order term in the displacement field perturbations that are due to the presence of a small volume anomaly.

7.6 Nearly Incompressible Bodies

We formally establish an asymptotic development of the solution to (7.15) as λ and $\tilde{\lambda}$ go to $+\infty$ with $\tilde{\lambda}/\lambda$ of order one. We find that the displacement field $\mathbf{u}$ can be represented in the form of a power series:

$$\mathbf{u} = \mathbf{u}_0 + (\frac{1}{\lambda}\chi(\Omega \setminus D) + \frac{1}{\tilde{\lambda}}\chi(D))\,\mathbf{u}_1 + (\frac{1}{\lambda^2}\chi(\Omega \setminus D) + \frac{1}{\tilde{\lambda}^2}\chi(D))\,\mathbf{u}_2 + \cdots,$$

where $\mathbf{u}_i$ for $i = 0, 1, \ldots$, are solutions to modified Stokes systems, the one used for computing the leading-order term $\mathbf{u}_0$ being homogeneous. It can be proven that this asymptotic series strongly converges in an appropriate Sobolev space.

Suppose for simplicity that $\int_{\partial\Omega} \mathbf{g} \cdot \mathbf{N} = 0$. Set

$$p := \begin{cases} \lambda\nabla \cdot \mathbf{u} & \text{in } \Omega \setminus \overline{D}, \\ \tilde{\lambda}\nabla \cdot \mathbf{u} & \text{in } D, \end{cases} \tag{7.32}$$

and rewrite (7.15) in the following form:

$$\begin{cases} \mu\Delta\mathbf{u} + (1 + \frac{\mu}{\lambda})\nabla p + \omega^2\mathbf{u} = 0 & \text{in } \Omega \setminus \overline{D}, \\ \tilde{\mu}\Delta\mathbf{u} + (1 + \frac{\tilde{\mu}}{\tilde{\lambda}})\nabla p + \omega^2\mathbf{u} = 0 & \text{in } D, \\ \mathbf{u}\big|_- = \mathbf{u}\big|_+ & \text{on } \partial D, \\ (p\mathbf{N} + \tilde{\mu}\frac{\partial\mathbf{u}}{\partial\mathbf{N}})\big|_- = (p\mathbf{N} + \mu\frac{\partial\mathbf{u}}{\partial\mathbf{N}})\big|_+ & \text{on } \partial D, \\ \mathbf{u}\big|_{\partial\Omega} = \mathbf{g}. \end{cases} \tag{7.33}$$

We look for a solution of (7.33) in the form of power series

$$\begin{cases} \mathbf{u} = \mathbf{u}_0 + (\frac{1}{\lambda}\chi(\Omega \setminus D) + \frac{1}{\tilde{\lambda}}\chi(D))\,\mathbf{u}_1 + (\frac{1}{\lambda^2}\chi(\Omega \setminus D) + \frac{1}{\tilde{\lambda}^2}\chi(D))\,\mathbf{u}_2 + \cdots, \\ p = p_0 + (\frac{1}{\lambda}\chi(\Omega \setminus D) + \frac{1}{\tilde{\lambda}}\chi(D))\,p_1 + (\frac{1}{\lambda^2}\chi(\Omega \setminus D) + \frac{1}{\tilde{\lambda}^2}\chi(D))\,p_2 + \cdots. \end{cases}$$

This leads to the recurrence relations

$$\begin{cases} (\mu\Delta + \omega^2)\mathbf{u}_0 + \nabla p_0 = 0 & \text{in } \Omega \setminus \overline{D}, \\ (\tilde{\mu}\Delta + \omega^2)\mathbf{u}_0 + \nabla p_0 = 0 & \text{in } D, \\ \mathbf{u}_0\big|_- = \mathbf{u}_0\big|_+ & \text{on } \partial D, \\ (p_0|_+ - p_0|_-)\mathbf{N} + \mu\frac{\partial\mathbf{u}_0}{\partial\mathbf{N}}\big|_+ - \tilde{\mu}\frac{\partial\mathbf{u}_0}{\partial\mathbf{N}}\big|_- = 0 & \text{on } \partial D, \\ \nabla \cdot \mathbf{u}_0 = 0 & \text{in } \Omega, \\ \mathbf{u}_0 = \mathbf{g} & \text{on } \partial\Omega, \\ \int_\Omega p_0 = 0, \end{cases} \tag{7.34}$$

and, for $j \geq 1$,

$$
\begin{cases}
(\mu\Delta + \omega^2)\mathbf{u}_j + \nabla p_j + \mu\nabla p_{j-1} = 0 & \text{in } \Omega \setminus \overline{D}, \\[4pt]
(\tilde{\mu}\Delta + \omega^2)\mathbf{u}_j + \nabla p_j + \tilde{\mu}\nabla p_{j-1} = 0 & \text{in } D, \\[4pt]
\mathbf{u}_j\big|_- = \left(\dfrac{\tilde{\lambda}}{\lambda}\right)^{j} \mathbf{u}_j\big|_+ & \text{on } \partial D, \\[6pt]
\left(\dfrac{\tilde{\lambda}}{\lambda}\right)^{j} \left(p_j\big|_+\mathbf{N} + \mu\dfrac{\partial\mathbf{u}_j}{\partial\mathbf{N}}\Big|_+\right) - \left(p_j\big|_-\mathbf{N} + \tilde{\mu}\dfrac{\partial\mathbf{u}_j}{\partial\mathbf{N}}\Big|_-\right) = 0 & \text{on } \partial D, \\[6pt]
\nabla \cdot \mathbf{u}_j = p_{j-1} & \text{in } \Omega, \\[4pt]
\mathbf{u}_j = 0 & \text{on } \partial\Omega, \\[4pt]
\displaystyle\int_\Omega p_j = 0.
\end{cases}
\tag{7.35}
$$

Equations (7.34) are the time-harmonic linearized equations of incompressible fluids or the modified Stokes system. Equations (7.35) are nonhomogeneous.

Suppose that the anomaly $D = \delta B + z$. We derive the leading-order term in the asymptotic expansion of $\mathbf{u}_0$ as δ goes to zero.

7.6.1 Formal Derivations

We give a formal derivation of the leading-order term in the asymptotic expansion of $\mathbf{u}_0$ as $\delta \to 0$. Let $(\mathbf{U}_0, q_0)$ denote the background solution to the modified Stokes system (7.36), that is, the solution to

$$
\begin{cases}
(\mu\Delta + \omega^2)\mathbf{U}_0 + \nabla q_0 = 0 & \text{in } \Omega, \\[4pt]
\nabla \cdot \mathbf{U}_0 = 0 & \text{in } \Omega, \\[4pt]
\mathbf{U}_0 = \mathbf{g} & \text{on } \partial\Omega, \\[4pt]
\displaystyle\int_\Omega q_0 = 0.
\end{cases}
\tag{7.36}
$$

Note that if $\mathbf{U}$ is a shear wave (i.e. divergence-free) then $q_0 = 0$.

We introduce the local variables $\xi = (y - z)/\delta$ for $y \in \Omega$, and set $\hat{\mathbf{u}}_0(\xi) = \mathbf{u}_0(z + \delta\xi)$. We expect again that $\mathbf{u}_0(y)$ will differ appreciably from $\mathbf{U}_0(y)$ for y near z, but it will differ little from $\mathbf{U}_0(y)$ for y far from z. Therefore, we shall represent the field $\mathbf{u}_0$ (and p_0) by two different expansions, an inner expansion for y near z, and an outer expansion for y far from z. The outer expansion must begin with $\mathbf{U}_0$ (respectively q_0), so we write:

$$
\begin{aligned}
\mathbf{u}_0(y) &= \mathbf{U}_0(y) + \delta^{\tau_1}\mathbf{U}_1(y) + \delta^{\tau_2}\mathbf{U}_2(y) + \dots, \\
p_0(y) &= q_0(y) + \delta^{\tau_1}q_1(y) + \delta^{\tau_2}q_2(y) + \dots, \quad \text{for } |y - z| \gg O(\delta),
\end{aligned}
$$

where $0 < \tau_1 < \tau_2 < \dots$, $\mathbf{U}_1, \mathbf{U}_2, \dots$, and $q_1, q_2, \dots$, are to be found.

We write the inner expansion as

$$\hat{\mathbf{u}}_0(\xi) = \mathbf{u}_0(z + \delta\xi) = \hat{\mathbf{v}}_0(\xi) + \delta\hat{\mathbf{v}}_1(\xi) + \delta^2\hat{\mathbf{v}}_2(\xi) + \dots ,$$
$$\hat{p}_0(\xi) = p_0(z + \delta\xi) = \hat{p}_0(\xi) + \delta\hat{p}_1(\xi) + \delta^2\hat{p}_2(\xi) + \dots , \quad \text{for } |\xi| = O(1) ,$$

where $\hat{\mathbf{v}}_0, \hat{\mathbf{v}}_1, \dots$, are to be found. We assume that the functions $\hat{\mathbf{v}}_j, j = 0, 1, \dots$, are defined not just in the domain obtained by stretching Ω, but everywhere in $\mathbb{R}^3$.

In order to determine the functions $\mathbf{U}_i(y), q_i(y)$ and $\hat{\mathbf{v}}_i(\xi), \hat{p}_i(\xi)$, we have to equate the inner and the outer expansions in some overlap domain within which the stretched variable ξ is large and $y - z$ is small. In this domain the matching conditions are:

$$\mathbf{U}_0(y) + \delta^{\tau_1}\mathbf{U}_1(y) + \delta^{\tau_2}\mathbf{U}_2(y) + \dots \sim \hat{\mathbf{v}}_0(\xi) + \delta\hat{\mathbf{v}}_1(\xi) + \delta^2\hat{\mathbf{v}}_2(\xi) + \dots$$

and

$$q_0(y) + \delta^{\tau_1}q_1(y) + \delta^{\tau_2}q_2(y) + \dots \sim \hat{p}_0(\xi) + \delta\hat{p}_1(\xi) + \delta^2\hat{p}_2(\xi) + \dots .$$

If we substitute the inner expansion into the transmission problem (7.34) and formally equate coefficients of δ^{-2}, δ^{-1} we get: $\hat{\mathbf{v}}_0(\xi) = \mathbf{U}_0(z)$, and

$$\begin{cases} \mu\Delta\hat{\mathbf{v}}_1 + \nabla\hat{p}_0 = 0 & \text{in } \mathbb{R}^3 \setminus \overline{B} , \\ \tilde{\mu}\Delta\hat{\mathbf{v}}_1 + \nabla\hat{p}_0 = 0 & \text{in } B , \\ \hat{\mathbf{v}}_1|_- - \hat{\mathbf{v}}_1|_+ = 0 & \text{on } \partial B , \\ (\hat{p}_0\mathbf{N} + \tilde{\mu}\dfrac{\partial\hat{\mathbf{v}}_1}{\partial\mathbf{N}})|_- - (\hat{p}_0\mathbf{N} + \mu\dfrac{\partial\hat{\mathbf{v}}_1}{\partial\mathbf{N}})|_+ = 0 & \text{on } \partial B , \\ \nabla\cdot\hat{\mathbf{v}}_1 = 0 & \text{in } \mathbb{R}^3 , \\ \hat{\mathbf{v}}_1(\xi) \to \nabla\mathbf{U}_0(z)\xi & \text{as } |\xi| \to +\infty , \\ \hat{p}_0(\xi) \to 0 & \text{as } |\xi| \to +\infty . \end{cases} \quad (7.37)$$

Therefore, we arrive at the following (inner) asymptotic formula:

$$\mathbf{u}_0(x) \approx \mathbf{U}_0(z) + \delta\hat{\mathbf{v}}_1(\frac{x - z}{\delta}) \quad \text{for } x \text{ near } z . \quad (7.38)$$

Note that $\nabla_\xi \cdot (\nabla\mathbf{U}_0(z)\xi) = \nabla\cdot\mathbf{U}_0(z) = 0$ in $\mathbb{R}^3$. Furthermore, we can prove that $\hat{\mathbf{v}}_1$ admits the following representation

$$\hat{\mathbf{v}}_1(\xi) = \begin{cases} \nabla\mathbf{U}_0(z)\xi + \mathcal{S}_B^0[\hat{\psi}](\xi) & \text{in } \mathbb{R}^3 \setminus \overline{B} , \\ \mathcal{S}_B^0[\hat{\phi}](\xi) & \text{in } B , \end{cases} \quad (7.39)$$

where $(\hat{\phi}, \hat{\psi})$ is the unique solution to

$$\begin{cases} \mathcal{S}_B^0[\hat{\phi}] - \mathcal{S}_B^0[\hat{\psi}] = \nabla\mathbf{U}_0(z)\xi & \text{on } \partial B , \\ \tilde{\mu}(-\dfrac{1}{2} + (\mathcal{K}_B^0)^*)[\hat{\phi}] - \mu(\dfrac{1}{2} + (\mathcal{K}_B^0)^*)[\hat{\psi}] = \dfrac{\partial}{\partial n}(\nabla\mathbf{U}_0(z)\xi) & \text{on } \partial B . \end{cases} \quad (7.40)$$

We now derive the outer expansion. Recall that $k_T = \omega/\sqrt{\mu}$. One can see from (7.34) and (7.36) that $(\mathbf{u}_0 - \mathbf{U}_0, p_0 - q_0)$ satisfies

$$
\begin{cases}
(\Delta + k_T^2)(\mathbf{u}_0 - \mathbf{U}_0) + \dfrac{1}{\mu}\nabla(p_0 - q_0) = 0 \quad \text{in } \Omega \setminus \overline{D}, \\[2mm]
(\Delta + k_T^2)(\mathbf{u}_0 - \mathbf{U}_0) + \dfrac{1}{\mu}\nabla(p_0 - q_0) = (k_T^2 - \tilde{k}_T^2)\mathbf{u}_0 \\[2mm]
\qquad\qquad + \left(\dfrac{1}{\mu} - \dfrac{1}{\tilde{\mu}}\right)\nabla p_0 \quad \text{in } D, \\[2mm]
(\mathbf{u}_0 - \mathbf{U}_0)\big|_+ - (\mathbf{u}_0 - \mathbf{U}_0)\big|_- = 0 \quad \text{on } \partial D, \\[2mm]
\dfrac{1}{\mu}(p_0 - q_0)\big|_+ \mathbf{N} + \dfrac{\partial}{\partial \mathbf{N}}(\mathbf{u}_0 - \mathbf{U}_0)\big|_+ = \dfrac{1}{\mu}(p_0 - q_0)\big|_- \mathbf{N} \\[2mm]
\qquad + \dfrac{\partial}{\partial \mathbf{N}}(\mathbf{u}_0 - \mathbf{U}_0)\big|_- + \dfrac{\tilde{\mu} - \mu}{\mu}\dfrac{\partial \mathbf{u}_0}{\partial \mathbf{N}}\bigg|_- \quad \text{on } \partial D, \\[2mm]
\nabla \cdot (\mathbf{u}_0 - \mathbf{U}_0) = 0 \quad \text{in } \Omega, \\[2mm]
\mathbf{u}_0 - \mathbf{U}_0 = 0 \quad \text{on } \partial \Omega.
\end{cases}
\tag{7.41}
$$

Integrating the first equation in (7.41) against the Green function $\mathbf{\Gamma}^{k_T}(x, y)$ over $y \in \Omega \setminus \overline{D}$ and using the divergence theorem, we obtain the following representation formula for $x \in \Omega$:

$$
\mathbf{u}_0(x) = \mathbf{U}_0(x) + \left(\dfrac{\tilde{\mu}}{\mu} - 1\right)\int_{\partial D} \mathbf{\Gamma}^{k_T}(x, y)\dfrac{\partial \mathbf{u}_0}{\partial \mathbf{N}}\big|_-(y)\, d\sigma(y)
$$
$$
+ \left(\dfrac{1}{\mu} - \dfrac{1}{\tilde{\mu}}\right)\int_D \mathbf{\Gamma}^{k_T}(x, y)\nabla p_0(y)\, dy + \omega^2\left(\dfrac{1}{\mu} - \dfrac{1}{\tilde{\mu}}\right)\int_D \mathbf{\Gamma}^{k_T}(x, y)\mathbf{u}_0(y)\, dy.
$$

Since

$$
\int_{\partial D} \dfrac{\partial \mathbf{u}_0}{\partial \mathbf{N}}\big|_-(y)\, d\sigma(y) + \dfrac{1}{\tilde{\mu}}\int_D \nabla p_0(y)\, dy = -\tilde{k}_T^2\int_D \mathbf{u}_0\, dy,
$$

as can be seen by integration by parts, we obtain from the inner expansion that for x far away from z,

$$
\mathbf{u}_0(x) \approx \mathbf{U}_0(x) + \delta^3 \sum_{i,j,\ell=1}^3 \mathbf{e}_i \partial_\ell G_{ij}^{k_T}(x, z)\bigg[\left(\dfrac{\tilde{\mu}}{\mu} - 1\right)\int_{\partial B}\left(\dfrac{\partial \hat{\mathbf{v}}_1}{\partial \mathbf{N}}\right)_j\bigg|_-(\xi)\xi_\ell\, d\sigma(\xi)
$$
$$
+ \left(\dfrac{1}{\mu} - \dfrac{1}{\tilde{\mu}}\right)\int_B \partial_j \hat{p}_0(\xi)\xi_\ell\, d\xi\bigg],
$$

where $(\partial \hat{\mathbf{v}}_1/\partial \mathbf{N})_j$ is the j-th component of $\partial \hat{\mathbf{v}}_1/\partial \mathbf{N}$, which we may simplify as follows

$$
\mathbf{u}_0 - \mathbf{U}_0 \approx \delta^3\left(\dfrac{\tilde{\mu}}{\mu} - 1\right)\sum_{i,j,\ell=1}^3 \mathbf{e}_i \partial_\ell G_{ij}^{k_T}(\cdot, z)\int_B (\partial_j \hat{\mathbf{v}}_{1\ell} + \partial_\ell \hat{\mathbf{v}}_{1j})(\xi)\, d\xi.
\tag{7.42}
$$

Here $\hat{\mathbf{v}}_{1j}$ denotes the j-th component of $\hat{\mathbf{v}}_1$.

Formulae (7.38) and (7.42) are formally derived asymptotic inner and outer expansions. They can be rigorously proven using layer potential techniques.

7.6.2 Viscous Moment Tensor

Let $d(\xi) := (1/3) \sum_k \xi_k \mathbf{e}_k$ and $\hat{\mathbf{v}}_{pq}$, for $p, q = 1, 2, 3$, be the solution to

$$
\begin{cases}
\mu \Delta \hat{\mathbf{v}}_{pq} + \nabla \hat{p} = 0 & \text{in } \mathbb{R}^3 \setminus \overline{B} , \\
\tilde{\mu} \Delta \hat{\mathbf{v}}_{pq} + \nabla \hat{p} = 0 & \text{in } B , \\
\hat{\mathbf{v}}_{pq}|_- - \hat{\mathbf{v}}_{pq}|_+ = 0 & \text{on } \partial B , \\
(\hat{p}\mathbf{N} + \tilde{\mu} \frac{\partial \hat{\mathbf{v}}_{pq}}{\partial \mathbf{N}})|_- - (\hat{p}\mathbf{N} + \mu \frac{\partial \hat{\mathbf{v}}_{pq}}{\partial \mathbf{N}})|_+ = 0 & \text{on } \partial B , \\
\nabla \cdot \hat{\mathbf{v}}_{pq} = 0 & \text{in } \mathbb{R}^3 , \\
\hat{\mathbf{v}}_{pq}(\xi) \to \xi_p \mathbf{e}_q - \delta_{pq} d(\xi) & \text{as } |\xi| \to \infty , \\
\hat{p}(\xi) \to 0 & \text{as } |\xi| \to +\infty .
\end{cases}
\tag{7.43}
$$

We define the viscous moment tensor (VMT) $(V_{ij}^{pq})_{i,j,p,q=1,2,3}$ by

$$
V_{ij}^{pq} = (\tilde{\mu} - \mu) \int_B \nabla \hat{\mathbf{v}}_{pq} \cdot (\nabla(\xi_i \mathbf{e}_j) + \nabla(\xi_i \mathbf{e}_j)^T) \, d\xi .
\tag{7.44}
$$

It is worth mentioning that the notion of a VMT can be defined in the same manner for two dimensions.

We will realize the notion of a VMT as a limit of the corresponding notion for the elasticity, the EMT, from which all the important properties of VMT will immediately follow. Before doing that, we rewrite (7.38) and (7.42) using the VMT.

Since $\mathbf{U}_0$ is divergence-free, we have

$$
\nabla \mathbf{U}_0(z)\xi = \sum_{p,q} \partial_q \mathbf{U}_0(z)_p (\xi_p \mathbf{e}_q - \delta_{pq} d(\xi)) ,
$$

and hence

$$
\hat{\mathbf{v}}_1 = \sum_{p,q=1}^3 \partial_q \mathbf{U}_0(z)_p \hat{\mathbf{v}}_{pq} .
$$

By (7.38) and (7.42), we have the following asymptotic expansions. Let $\hat{\mathbf{v}}_{pq}$ be the solution to (7.43). Then

$$
\mathbf{u}_0(x) \approx \mathbf{U}_0(z) + \delta \sum_{p,q=1}^3 \partial_q \mathbf{U}_0(z)_p \hat{\mathbf{v}}_{pq}\left(\frac{x-z}{\delta}\right) \quad \text{for } x \text{ near } z .
$$

Let (V_{ij}^{pq}) be the VMT defined by (7.44). The following expansion holds uniformly for $x \in \partial\Omega$:

$$
(\mathbf{u}_0 - \mathbf{U}_0)(x) \approx \delta^3 \left[\sum_{i,j,p,q,\ell=1}^3 \mathbf{e}_\ell \partial_j G_{\ell i}^{k_T}(x, z) \partial_q \mathbf{U}_0(z)_p V_{ij}^{pq} \right] .
\tag{7.45}
$$

The viscous moment tensor can also be defined using the layer potentials. Let $(\hat{\phi}_{pq}, \hat{\psi}_{pq})$ be the unique solution to the following system of equations on ∂B:

$$\begin{cases} \mathcal{S}_B^0[\hat{\phi}_{pq}] - \mathcal{S}_B^0[\hat{\psi}_{pq}] = \xi_p \mathbf{e}_q - \delta_{pq} d(\xi) \,, \\ \tilde{\mu}(-\dfrac{1}{2} + (\mathcal{K}_B^0)^*)[\hat{\phi}_{pq}] - \mu(\dfrac{1}{2} + (\mathcal{K}_B^0)^*)[\hat{\psi}_{pq}] = \dfrac{\partial}{\partial n}(\xi_p \mathbf{e}_q - \delta_{pq} d(\xi)) \,. \end{cases} \quad (7.46)$$

Then we have

$$\hat{\mathbf{v}}_{pq}(\xi) = \begin{cases} \xi_p \mathbf{e}_q - \delta_{pq} d(\xi) + \mathcal{S}_B^0[\hat{\psi}_{pq}](\xi) & \text{in } \mathbb{R}^3 \setminus \overline{B} \,, \\ \mathcal{S}_B^0[\hat{\phi}_{pq}](\xi) & \text{in } B \,. \end{cases} \quad (7.47)$$

Integrating by parts, and using (7.46), and (7.47), we have

$$V_{ij}^{pq} = (\tilde{\mu} - \mu) \int_B \nabla \hat{\mathbf{v}}_{pq} : (\nabla(\xi_i \mathbf{e}_j) + \nabla(\xi_i \mathbf{e}_j)^T)\, d\xi$$

$$= (\tilde{\mu} - \mu) \int_B \nabla \hat{\mathbf{v}}_{pq} : (\nabla(\xi_i \mathbf{e}_j - \delta_{ij} d(\xi)) + \nabla(\xi_i \mathbf{e}_j - \delta_{ij} d(\xi))^T)\, d\xi$$

$$= (\tilde{\mu} - \mu) \int_{\partial B} \hat{\mathbf{v}}_{pq} \cdot \frac{\partial}{\partial \mathbf{N}}(\xi_i \mathbf{e}_j - \delta_{ij} d(\xi))$$

$$= \int_{\partial B} \left(\tilde{\mu} \mathcal{S}_B^0[\hat{\phi}_{pq}] - \mu \mathcal{S}_B^0[\hat{\psi}_{pq}] - \mu \nabla(\xi_i \mathbf{e}_j - \delta_{ij} d(\xi)) \right) \cdot \frac{\partial}{\partial \mathbf{N}}(\xi_i \mathbf{e}_j - \delta_{ij} d(\xi))$$

$$= \int_{\partial B} \left(\tilde{\mu}(-\frac{1}{2} + (\mathcal{K}_B^0)^*)[\hat{\phi}_{pq}] - \mu(-\frac{1}{2} + (\mathcal{K}_B^0)^*)[\hat{\psi}_{pq}] \right.$$

$$\left. - \frac{\partial}{\partial n}(\xi_i \mathbf{e}_j - \delta_{ij} d(\xi)) \right) \cdot (\xi_i \mathbf{e}_j - \delta_{ij} d(\xi))$$

$$= \mu \int_{\partial B} \hat{\psi}_{pq} \cdot (\xi_i \mathbf{e}_j - \delta_{ij} d(\xi)) \,.$$

Therefore,

$$V_{ij}^{pq} = \mu \int_{\partial B} \hat{\psi}_{pq} \cdot (\xi_i \mathbf{e}_j - \delta_{ij} d(\xi)), \quad i,j,p,q = 1,2,3 \,, \quad (7.48)$$

where $(\hat{\phi}_{pq}, \hat{\psi}_{pq})$ is the unique solution to (7.46).

As the Stokes system appears as a limiting case of the Lamé system, there is a strong relation between VMT and EMT, which we give now.

Let $M = (m_{ij}^{pq})$ be the EMT associated with the domain B and the pairs of Lamé parameters (λ, μ) and $(\tilde{\lambda}, \tilde{\mu})$. We can prove that the following lemma holds.

Lemma 7.6.1 For $i,j,p,q = 1,2,3$,

$$V_{ij}^{pq} = \lim_{\lambda, \tilde{\lambda} \to \infty} \left(m_{ij}^{pq} - \frac{\delta_{ij}}{3}\sum_{k=1}^{3} m_{kk}^{pq} - \frac{\delta_{pq}}{3}\sum_{s=1}^{3} m_{ij}^{ss} + \frac{\delta_{ij}\delta_{pq}}{9}\sum_{k,s=1}^{3} m_{kk}^{ss} \right).$$

As an immediate consequence of Lemma 7.6.1 and the symmetry properties of the EMT, we have the following corollary.

Corollary 7.6.2 *For* $i, j, p, q = 1, 2, 3$,

$$V_{ij}^{pq} = V_{ji}^{pq}, \quad V_{ij}^{pq} = V_{ij}^{qp}, \quad V_{ij}^{pq} = V_{pq}^{ij} . \tag{7.49}$$

Moreover, the following holds:

$$\sum_p V_{ij}^{pp} = 0 \quad \text{for all } i, j \quad \text{and} \quad \sum_i V_{ii}^{pq} = 0 \quad \text{for all } p, q . \tag{7.50}$$

The relation in Lemma 7.6.1 has an interesting interpretation. The VMT V and the EMT M are 4-tensors and can be regarded as linear transformations on the space of symmetric matrices because of their symmetry. Recall that Λ_2 defined by (7.24) is the orthogonal projection from the space of symmetric matrices onto the space of symmetric matrices of trace zero. Then the relation in Lemma 7.6.1 is equivalent to

$$V = \lim_{\lambda, \tilde{\lambda} \to +\infty} \Lambda_2 M \Lambda_2 . \tag{7.51}$$

The formula (7.51) enables us to compute the VMT from the known formula of the EMT. For example, if B is a two dimensional disk, then we have from (7.51) and (7.25) that

$$V = 4 |B| \mu \frac{(\tilde{\mu} - \mu)}{\tilde{\mu} + \mu} \Lambda_2 .$$

Moreover, taking the limits of the bounds (7.28) and (7.30) as $\lambda, \tilde{\lambda} \to +\infty$ shows that in two dimensions $(1/(2\mu)) V$ satisfies the bounds

$$\frac{1}{(\frac{\tilde{\mu}}{\mu} - 1)} \mathrm{Tr}(\frac{1}{2\mu} V) \le |B|(1 + \frac{\mu}{\tilde{\mu}}) , \tag{7.52}$$

$$(\frac{\tilde{\mu}}{\mu} - 1) \mathrm{Tr}((\frac{1}{2\mu} V)^{-1}) \le \frac{1}{|B|}(1 + \frac{\tilde{\mu}}{\mu}) . \tag{7.53}$$

Note that, in view of Theorem 7.1.2, the right-hand sides of (7.52) and (7.53) are exactly the Hashin-Shtrikman bounds (7.9) for the PT associated with the same domain B and the conductivity contrast $k = \tilde{\mu}/\mu$.

7.7 Diffusion Equation

In optical tomography, the radiation transfer equation being an integro-differential equation, it leads to numerical problems of prohibited size unless simplifications are made. A common simplification, that is justified at least in the case of strongly scattering media, is the diffusion approximation. Assuming the speed of the light is constant in the medium, the diffusion approximation can be written as

$$
\begin{cases}
i\dfrac{\omega}{c}u - \nabla \cdot q\nabla u + \sigma u = 0 & \text{in } \Omega, \\[2mm]
q\dfrac{\partial u}{\partial \nu} = g & \text{on } \partial\Omega,
\end{cases}
\tag{7.54}
$$

where q is the diffusion coefficient, σ the absorption coefficient, c the presumably constant speed of light, and ω a given frequency.

Suppose that Ω contains a small anomaly of the form $D = \delta B + z$, as before. Denote by q_0 and σ_0 the diffusion coefficient and the absorption coefficient of the background medium Ω, and assume that $q_0 > 0$ and $\sigma_0 > 0$ are positive constants. Let $q_\star > 0$ and $\sigma_\star > 0$ denote the diffusion coefficient and the absorption coefficient of the anomaly D, which are also assumed to be positive constants.

In the exactly same manner as Theorem 7.2.1, we can prove that the following asymptotic formula holds.

Theorem 7.7.1 *If U denotes the background solution (in the absence of any anomalies) then, for any $x \in \partial\Omega$,*

$$
u(x) = U(x) - \delta^d \Big(\nabla U(z) M(\lambda, B) \nabla_z N(x, z)
$$

$$
+ (\sigma_\star - \sigma_0)|B|U(z)N(x, z) \Big) + O(\delta^{d+1}),
$$

where the Neumann function N is given by

$$
\begin{cases}
i\dfrac{\omega}{c}N(x, z) - q_0\Delta_x N(x, z) + \sigma_0 N(x, z) = \delta_z & \text{in } \Omega, \\[2mm]
\dfrac{\partial N}{\partial \nu_x} = 0 & \text{on } \partial\Omega,
\end{cases}
$$

and M the PT defined in (7.3) with λ given by

$$
\lambda := \frac{(q_\star/q_0) + 1}{2((q_\star/q_0) - 1)}.
$$

Bibliography and Discussion

Theorem 7.1.1 was proven in [61, 36, 12]. The results of Sect. 7.2 are from [120, 14]. The original Hashin-Shtrikman bounds can be found in the book by Milton [100]. The Hashin-Shtrikman bounds for the polarization tensor were proved in [92, 35]. Parts (i) and (ii) in Theorem 7.3.2 as well as Theorem 7.3.1 were established in [18]. The explicit formula for the EMT for an ellipse is from [17]. The bounds in part (iii) were obtained in [92, 33]. The results on the VMT are from [8]. The initial boundary-value problems for the (time-dependent) acoustic and elastic wave equations in the presence of anomalies of small volume have been considered in [3, 15]. In those papers, asymptotic formulae for the perturbations due to the anomalies for a finite interval in time are rigorously derived.

The optical tomography problem is discussed in the review paper [21]. A derivation of the diffusion approximation for the radiation transfer equation can be found in [74]. A high-order asymptotic expansion of the solution to the diffusion equation with an absorbing inclusion (with $q_\star = q_0$) of small volume is presented in [24].

Imaging Techniques

In this chapter we apply the accurate asymptotic formulae derived in Chap. 7 for the purpose of identifying the location and certain properties of the shape of the anomalies. We also discuss time-domain imaging of small anomalies. We restrict ourselves to conductivity and electromagnetic imaging and single out simple fundamental algorithms. Based on the asymptotic modeling in Sect. 7.4, these algorithms can be extended in the context of elastic imaging to detect the location and the EMT of a small elastic anomaly.

8.1 Projection Type Algorithms

The projection algorithm is a fast, stable, and efficient algorithm. It takes advantage of the smallness of the anomalies. For the sake of simplicity, we only consider the reconstruction of small conductivity anomalies. A similar algorithm to the one described here can be designed for imaging small elastic anomalies.

The method of finding conductivity anomalies is based on the asymptotic expansion formula (7.2). However, the formula (7.2) is expressed in terms of the Neumann function $N(x, z)$ which depends on the domain Ω. There is a trick to overcome this difficulty. For $g \in L_0^2(\partial\Omega)$, define the harmonic function $H[g](x)$, $x \in \mathbb{R}^d \setminus \overline{\Omega}$, by

$$H[g](x) := -\mathcal{S}_\Omega(g)(x) + \mathcal{D}_\Omega(u|_{\partial\Omega})(x) , \quad x \in \mathbb{R}^d \setminus \overline{\Omega} . \tag{8.1}$$

Since $-\mathcal{S}_\Omega(g)(x) + \mathcal{D}_\Omega(U|_{\partial\Omega})(x) = 0$ for $x \in \mathbb{R}^d \setminus \overline{\Omega}$, we have

$$H[g](x) = \mathcal{D}_\Omega(u|_{\partial\Omega} - U|_{\partial\Omega})(x) . \tag{8.2}$$

Then by using a simple formula $\mathcal{D}_\Omega(N(\cdot - z))(x) = \Gamma(x - z)$ for $z \in \Omega$ and $x \in \mathbb{R}^d \setminus \overline{\Omega}$, we get

$$H[g](x) = -\delta^d \partial U(z) M(\lambda, B) \partial_z \Gamma(x - z) + O(\delta^{d+1}) , \tag{8.3}$$

for all $x \in \mathbb{R}^d \setminus \overline{\Omega}$.

The projection algorithm makes use of constant current sources. We want to apply a special type of current that makes ∂U constant in D. Injection current $g = \mathbf{a} \cdot \nu$ for a fixed unit vector $\mathbf{a} \in \mathbb{R}^d$ yields $\nabla U = \mathbf{a}$ in Ω.

Let $H[\mathbf{a} \cdot \nu]$ denote the function H in (8.2) corresponding to the Neumann data $g = \mathbf{a} \cdot \nu$. Assume for the sake of simplicity that $d = 2$ and D is a disk. Then from (7.7) and (8.3), it follows that

$$H[\mathbf{a} \cdot \nu](x) \approx \frac{(k-1)|D|}{\pi(k+1)} \frac{(x-z) \cdot \mathbf{a}}{|x-z|^2} + O(\delta^3) , \quad x \in \mathbb{R}^2 \setminus \overline{\Omega} . \tag{8.4}$$

The first step for the reconstruction procedure is to locate the anomaly. The location search algorithm is as follows. Take two observation lines Σ_1 and Σ_2 contained in $\mathbb{R}^2 \setminus \overline{\Omega}$ given by

$$\Sigma_1 := \text{ a line parallel to } \mathbf{a} ,$$

$$\Sigma_2 := \text{ a line normal to } \mathbf{a} .$$

Find two points $P_i \in \Sigma_i, i = 1, 2$, so that

$$H[\mathbf{a} \cdot \nu](P_1) = 0, \quad H[\mathbf{a} \cdot \nu](P_2) = \max_{x \in \Sigma_2} |H[\mathbf{a} \cdot \nu](x)| .$$

From (8.4), we can see that the intersecting point P of the two lines

$$\{(x - P_1) \cdot \mathbf{a} = 0\} \quad \text{and} \quad \{(x - P_2) \cdot \mathbf{a}^\perp = 0\}$$

is close to the center z of the anomaly D.

Once we locate the anomaly, the factor $|D|(k-1)/(k+1)$ can be estimated. Note that this information is a mixture of the conductivity and the volume. It is impossible to extract the conductivity from the PT. A small anomaly with high conductivity and larger anomaly with lower conductivity can have the same PT.

An arbitrary shaped anomaly can be represented and visualized by means of an ellipse or an ellipsoid with the same polarization tensor. See Fig. 8.1.

8.2 Multiple Signal Classification Type Algorithms

The MUSIC algorithm is essentially a method of characterizing the range of a self-adjoint operator. Suppose A is a self-adjoint operator with eigenvalues $\lambda_1 \geq \lambda_2 \geq \ldots$ and corresponding eigenvectors $v_1, v_2, \ldots$. Suppose the eigenvalues $\lambda_{n+1}, \lambda_{n+2}, \ldots$ are all zero, so that the vectors $v_{n+1}, v_{n+2}, \ldots$ span the null space of A. Alternatively, $\lambda_{n+1}, \lambda_{n+2}, \ldots$ could merely be very small, below the noise level of the system represented by A; in this case we say that the vectors $v_{n+1}, v_{n+2}, \ldots$ span the noise subspace of A. We can form the projection onto the noise subspace; this projection is given explicitly by

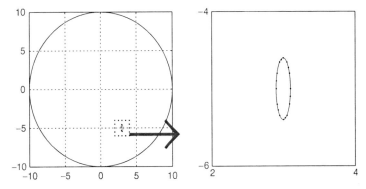

Fig. 8.1. Detection of the location and the polarization tensor of a small arbitrary shaped anomaly by a projection type algorithm. The shape of the anomaly is approximated by an ellipse with the same polarization tensor.

$P_{\text{noise}} = \sum_{p>n} v_p \overline{v_p}^T$, where the subscript T denotes the transpose and the bar denotes the complex conjugate. The (essential) range of A, meanwhile, is spanned by the vectors $v_1, v_2, \dots, v_n$.

The key idea of MUSIC is this: because A is self-adjoint, we know that the noise subspace is orthogonal to the (essential) range. Therefore, a vector f is in the range of A if and only if its projection onto the noise subspace is zero, *i.e.*, if $\|P_{\text{noise}} f\| = 0$, or equivalently,

$$\frac{1}{\|P_{\text{noise}} f\|} = +\infty \,. \tag{8.5}$$

Equation (8.5) is the MUSIC characterization of the range of A. If A is not self-adjoint, MUSIC can be used with the singular-value decomposition (SVD) instead of the eigenvalue decomposition.

MUSIC is generally used in signal processing problems as a method for estimating the individual frequencies of multiple time-harmonic signals.

In this section we apply the MUSIC algorithm to determine the locations of several small electromagnetic anomalies.

Suppose that an electromagnetic medium occupies a bounded domain Ω in $\mathbb{R}^d$, with a connected $\mathcal{C}^2$-boundary $\partial\Omega$. Suppose that Ω contains a finite number of well-separated small anomalies, each of the form $D_s = \delta B_s + z_s$, where $z_s \in \Omega$ and B_s is a $\mathcal{C}^2$-bounded domain in $\mathbb{R}^d$ containing the origin.

Let μ_0 and ε_0 denote the magnetic permeability and the electric permittivity of the background medium Ω, and assume that $\mu_0 > 0$ and $\varepsilon_0 > 0$ are positive constants. Let $\mu_s > 0$ and $\varepsilon_s > 0$ denote the permeability and the permittivity of the anomaly D_s, which are also assumed to be positive constants. Introduce the piecewise-constant magnetic permeability

$$\mu_\delta(x) = \begin{cases} \mu_0 \,, & x \in \Omega \setminus \overline{\cup_s D_s} \,, \\ \mu_s \,, & x \in D_s, s = 1, \dots, m \,, \end{cases}$$

and define the piecewise constant electric permittivity, $\varepsilon_\delta(x)$, analogously.

Let the electric field u denote the solution to the Helmholtz equation

$$\nabla \cdot \left(\frac{1}{\mu_\delta}\nabla u\right) + \omega^2 \varepsilon_\delta u = 0 \quad \text{in } \Omega ,$$

with the boundary condition $u = f \in W_{\frac{1}{2}}^2(\partial\Omega)$, where $\omega > 0$ the operating frequency. Assume that (7.11) holds. Since the anomalies are well-separated, it follows from (7.12) that the following asymptotic formula holds. For any $x \in \partial\Omega$,

$$\frac{\partial u}{\partial \nu}(x) = \frac{\partial U}{\partial \nu}(x) + \delta^d \sum_{s=1}^m \left(\nabla U(z_s) M(\lambda_s, B_s)\frac{\partial \nabla_z G_{k_0}(x, z_s)}{\partial \nu_x}\right.$$

$$\left. + \omega^2 \mu_0(\varepsilon_s - \varepsilon_0)|B_s|U(z_s)\frac{\partial G_{k_0}(x, z_s)}{\partial \nu_x}\right) + O(\delta^{d+1}) ,$$

where $M(\lambda_s, B_s)$ is the polarization tensor defined in (7.3) with λ_s given by

$$\lambda_s := \frac{(\mu_0/\mu_s) + 1}{2((\mu_0/\mu_s) - 1)} .$$

Therefore, for any smooth function V satisfying $(\Delta + k_0^2)V = 0$ in $\overline{\Omega}$, we have

$$\int_{\partial\Omega}\left(\frac{\partial u}{\partial \nu} - \frac{\partial U}{\partial \nu}\right)(x)V(x)\,d\sigma(x) \approx \delta^d \sum_{s=1}^m \left(\nabla U(z_s) M(\lambda_s, B_s)\nabla V(z_s)\right.$$

$$\left. + \omega^2 \mu_0(\varepsilon_s - \varepsilon_0)|B_s|U(z_s)V(z_s)\right) .$$

Let $(\theta_1,\ldots,\theta_n)$ be n unit vectors in $\mathbb{R}^d$. For arbitrary $\theta \in \{\theta_1,\ldots,\theta_n\}$, one assumes that one is in possession of the boundary data $\partial u/\partial \nu$ when the object Ω is illuminated with the plane wave $U(x) = e^{ik_0\theta\cdot x}$. Therefore, taking $V(x) = e^{ik_0\theta'\cdot x}$ for $\theta' \in \{\theta_1,\ldots,\theta_n\}$, shows that we are in possession of

$$\delta^d k_0^2 \sum_{s=1}^m \left(-\theta^T \cdot M(\lambda_s, B_s)\cdot\theta' + \left(\frac{\varepsilon_s}{\varepsilon_0} - 1\right)|B_s|\right)e^{ik_0(\theta+\theta')\cdot z_s} ,$$

for $\theta, \theta' \in \{\theta_1,\ldots,\theta_n\}$. Define the matrix $A = (A_{ll'})_{l,l'=1}^n \in \mathbb{C}^{n\times n}$ by

$$A_{ll'} = \sum_{s=1}^m \left(\theta_l^T \cdot M^s \cdot \theta_{l'} + \left(1 - \frac{\varepsilon_s}{\varepsilon_0}\right)|B_s|\right)e^{ik_0(\theta_l+\theta_{l'})\cdot z_s}, \quad l, l' = 1,\ldots,n ,$$

where $M^s := M(\lambda_s, B_s)$. Introduce the notation

$$v_s = \left((1,\theta_1)^T e^{ik_0\theta_1\cdot z_s},\ldots,(1,\theta_n)^T e^{ik_0\theta_n\cdot z_s}\right)^T$$

to rewrite the matrix A as a sum of outer products:

$$A = \sum_{s=1}^{m} v_s \begin{pmatrix} (1 - \frac{\varepsilon_s}{\varepsilon_0})|B_s| & 0 \\ 0 & M^s \end{pmatrix} v_s^T .$$

Our matrix A, called the multi-static response matrix (MSR), is symmetric, but it is not Hermitian. We form a Hermitian matrix $\widetilde{A} = \overline{A}A$. We note that $\overline{A}$ is the frequency-domain version of a time-reversed multi-static response matrix; thus $\widetilde{A}$ corresponds to performing an experiment, time-reversing the received signals and using them as input for a second experiment. The matrix $\widetilde{A}$ can be written as follows

$$\widetilde{A} = \sum_{s=1}^{m} \overline{v_s} \begin{pmatrix} (1 - \frac{\varepsilon_s}{\varepsilon_0})|B_s| & 0 \\ 0 & M^s \end{pmatrix} \overline{v_s}^T \sum_{s=1}^{m} v_s \begin{pmatrix} (1 - \frac{\varepsilon_s}{\varepsilon_0})|B_s| & 0 \\ 0 & M^s \end{pmatrix} v_s^T .$$

For any point $z \in \Omega$ we define g_z by

$$g_z = \left((1, \theta_1)^T e^{ik_0\theta_1 \cdot z}, \ldots, (1, \theta_n)^T e^{ik_0\theta_n \cdot z} \right)^T .$$

It can be shown that there exists $n_0 \in \mathbb{N}, n_0 > (d+1)m$, such that for any $n \geq n_0$ the following statement holds:

$$g_z \in \text{Range}(\widetilde{A}) \text{ if and only if } z \in \{z_1, \ldots, z_m\} .$$

The MUSIC algorithm can now be used as follows to determine the location of the anomalies. Let $P_{\text{noise}} = I - P$, where P is the orthogonal projection onto the range of $\widetilde{A}$. Given any point $z \in \Omega$, form the vector g_z. The point z coincides with the location of an anomaly if and only if $P_{\text{noise}}g_z = 0$. Thus we can form an image of the anomalies by plotting, at each point z, the cost function $1/\|P_{\text{noise}}g_z\|$. The resulting plot will have large peaks at the locations of the anomalies. See Fig. 8.3.

As pointed out the eigenvectors of the Hermitian matrix $\widetilde{A}$ can be computed by the SVD of the response matrix A. The eigenvalues of $\widetilde{A}$ are the squares of the singular values of A. An immediate application of the SVD of A is the determination of the number of anomalies. If, for example, $\mu_s \neq \mu_0$ and $\varepsilon_s \neq \varepsilon_0$ for all $s = 1, \ldots, m$, then there are exactly $(d+1)m$ significant singular values of A and the rest are zero or close to zero. If therefore the SVD of A has no significant singular values, then there are no detectable anomalies in the medium. Now, when there are detectable anomalies in the medium, we can use the eigenvectors corresponding to significant eigenvalues to locate them since these vectors span the range of $\widetilde{A}$. The eigenvectors corresponding to significant eigenvalues span some kind of signal subspace in the sense that they contain nearly all the information about the inclusions which can be extracted from the MSR matrix. The others span some kind of noise subspace. See Fig. 8.2.

The significant singular values of A can be used to estimate $((\varepsilon_s/\varepsilon_0) - 1)|D|$ and the eigenvalues of $\delta^d M^s$. To illustrate this, let us for simplicity consider the two-dimensional case and assume that there is only one anomaly of circular shape in the background, *i.e.* $m = 1$. From the boundary data $\partial u/\partial \nu$ corresponding to the illumination in the θ-direction of the object Ω with the plane wave

$$U(x) = e^{ik_0\theta \cdot x}, \quad \theta \in \{\theta_1, \ldots, \theta_n\},$$

we can reconstruct the coefficients

$$((\varepsilon_1/\varepsilon_0) - 1)|D| \quad \text{and} \quad 2|D|k_0^2(\mu_1 - \mu_0)/(\mu_1 + \mu_0)$$

as the singular values of the matrix $-\delta^2 k_0^2 A$, the second one being with multiplicity two.

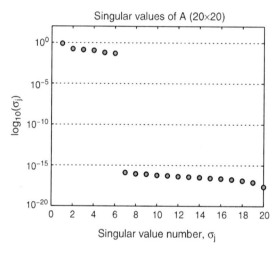

Fig. 8.2. SVD of the muti-static response matrix A corresponding to two well-separated electromagnetic anomalies of general shape for $n = 20$, using a standard log scale. 6 singular values emerge from the 14 others in the noise subspace.

Based on the asymptotic modeling in Sect. 7.4, our MUSIC-type algorithm can be extended to elastic imaging. Again, it yields a fast numbering, accurate localization, and optimal estimates of the elastic and geometric (elastic moment tensors) of the anomalies from a singular value decomposition of the corresponding MSR matrix.

8.3 Time-Domain Imaging

In this section, we briefly discuss some promising techniques for imaging small anomalies in the time-domain. As with time-independent problems, asymptotic expansions are derived for the purpose of identifying the location and

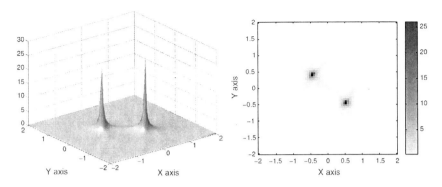

Fig. 8.3. MUSIC type reconstruction from the SVD of A represented in Fig. 8.2.

certain properties of the shape of the anomalies from measurements in the time-domain. Two classes of imaging techniques are described: (i) Fourier and MUSIC-type algorithms based on weighted asymptotic formulae and (ii) a time-reversal approach based on a pointwise asymptotic formula together with the spatial reciprocity and the time reversal invariance of the wave equation.

8.3.1 Fourier- and MUSIC-Type Algorithms

Let T_f be a final observation time, $\Omega_{T_f} = \Omega\times]0, T_f[$, $\partial\Omega_{T_f} = \partial\Omega\times]0, T_f[$, and $u_1 \in L^2(\Omega)$. Suppose that the Neumann boundary data $g \in \mathcal{C}^0(0, T_f; L^2(\partial\Omega))$ and the initial data $u_0 \in W^{1,2}(\Omega)$ are subject to the compatibility condition

$$\frac{\partial u_0}{\partial \nu} = g(\cdot, 0) \quad \text{on } \partial\Omega .$$

Consider the initial boundary value problem for the wave equation

$$\begin{cases} \partial_t^2 u - \nabla \cdot \left(\chi(\Omega \setminus \overline{D}) + k\chi(D) \right)\nabla u = 0 & \text{in} \quad \Omega_{T_f} , \\ u(x,0) = u_0(x), \quad \partial_t u(x,0) = u_1(x) & \text{for} \quad x \in \Omega , \\ \dfrac{\partial u}{\partial \nu} = g \quad \text{on} \quad \partial\Omega_{T_f} . \end{cases} \tag{8.6}$$

Define the background solution U to be the solution of the wave equation in the absence of any anomalies. Thus U satisfies

$$\begin{cases} \partial_t^2 U - \Delta U = 0 & \text{in} \quad \Omega_{T_f} , \\ U(x,0) = u_0(x), \quad \partial_t U(x,0) = u_1(x) & \text{for} \quad x \in \Omega , \\ \dfrac{\partial U}{\partial \nu} = g \quad \text{on} \quad \partial\Omega_{T_f} . \end{cases}$$

The following asymptotic expansion of weighted boundary measurements holds as $\delta \to 0$.

Theorem 8.3.1 (Weighted Boundary Measurements) *Let* $w \in C^\infty$ $(\overline{\Omega}_{T_f})$ *satisfy* $(\partial_t^2 - \Delta)w(x,t) = 0$ *in* Ω_{T_f} *with* $\partial_t w(x, T_f) = w(x, T_f) = 0$ *for* $x \in \Omega$. *Define the weighted boundary measurements*

$$I_w(T_f) := \int_{\partial\Omega_{T_f}} (u - U)(x,t)\frac{\partial w}{\partial \nu}(x,t)\, d\sigma(x)\, dt \ .$$

Then, for any fixed $T_f > \mathrm{diam}(\Omega)$, *the following asymptotic expansion for* $I_w(T_f)$ *holds as* $\delta \to 0$:

$$I_w(T_f) \approx \delta^d \int_0^{T_f} \nabla U(z,t) M(k,B) \nabla w(z,t)\, dt \ , \tag{8.7}$$

where $M(k,B)$ *is defined by (7.3).*

Let θ and θ' be two vectors in $\mathbb{R}^d$ such that $|\theta| = |\theta'|$. Choose the w to be the Dirac function at $t = x \cdot \theta/|\theta|$ and U to be a plane wave:

$$w(x,t) = \delta_{t=x\cdot\theta/|\theta|} \quad \text{and} \quad U(x,t) = e^{i(\theta'\cdot x + |\theta'|t)} \ .$$

With the notation of Sect. 8.2, the asymptotic expansion (8.7) yields

$$I(\theta,\theta') := I_w(T_f) \approx i\delta^d \sum_{s=1}^m \theta M(k_s, B_s)\theta' e^{i(\theta+\theta')\cdot z_s} \ ,$$

where z_s for $s = 1,\ldots,m$, are the locations of the conductivity anomalies $D_s = z_s + \delta B_s$ that have conductivities $k_s \neq 1$.

Based on Theorem 8.3.1 we propose the following three direct algorithms. The first and second algorithms are of Fourier type while the third one is of MUSIC type.

Let $r > 0$ and let $(\theta_1,\ldots,\theta_n)$ be n vectors in S_r, where S_r denotes the $(d-1)$-sphere of radius r which is centered at the origin. Suppose that we are in possession of $I(\theta,\theta')$ for $\theta,\theta' \in (\theta_1,\ldots,\theta_n)$.

First algorithm: Suppose that $\theta = \theta'$. Suppose that r takes values $r_0 = 0 <$ $r_1 < \ldots < r_p = R$. Then, applying Shannon's sampling theorem 2.3.1, a numerical discrete fast Fourier inversion of a sample of $I(\theta,\theta)$ will yield the locations z_s with a spatial resolution of order $2\pi/R$ as δ goes to zero.

Second algorithm: Since any vector $\zeta \in B_{2r}$, where B_{2r} is the ball of radius $2r$ centered at the origin, can be written as the sum of two vectors θ and $\theta' \in S_r$, then defining $I(\zeta) := I(\theta,\theta')$ for $\zeta = \theta + \theta'$, a numerical discrete fast Fourier inversion of a sample of $I(\zeta)$ will yield the locations z_s with a spatial resolution of order π/r as δ goes to zero.

Third algorithm: Fix $r > 0$. Consider the response matrix $A = (A_{ll'})_{l,l'=1}^n$, where $A_{ll'} = I(\theta_l, \theta_{l'})$. Let

$$g_z = \left(\theta_1^T e^{i\theta_1 \cdot z}, \ldots, \theta_n^T e^{i\theta_n \cdot z} \right)^T \ .$$

We can prove that

$$g_z \in \text{Range}\ (A) \quad \text{if and only if}\quad z \in \{z_1, \ldots, z_m\}\ .$$

As with the Helmholtz equation, the MUSIC algorithm is as follows. Denote P_{noise} the orthogonal projection onto the left null space (noise space) of the matrix A. We can form an image of the locations, $z_1, \ldots, z_m$, by plotting, at each point z, the quantity $1/\|P_{\text{noise}}g_z\|$. The operator P_{noise} is computed via a singular value decomposition of the matrix A.

8.3.2 Time-Reversal Imaging

We shall present the time-reversal method in the context of imaging small conductivity anomalies. The main idea of time-reversal is to take advantage of the reversibility of the wave equation in a non-dissipative unknown medium to back-propagate signals to the sources that emitted them.

For the sake of simplicity, we only consider the three-dimensional problem but stress that the time-reversal imaging discussed here applies directly to problems in two dimensions. The derivations in this section are formal.

Asymptotic Formula

Let $y \in \mathbb{R}^3$ be such that $|y - z| \gg \delta$. Set

$$U(x,t) := U_y(x,t) := \frac{\delta_{t=|x-y|}}{4\pi|x-y|} \quad \text{for } x \neq y\ . \tag{8.8}$$

U_y is a fundamental solution to the wave equation. It satisfies

$$(\partial_t^2 - \Delta)U_y(x,t) = \delta_{x=y}\delta_{t=0} \quad \text{in } \mathbb{R}^3 \times]0, +\infty[\ ,$$

in the sense of distributions, together with the initial conditions:

$$U_y(x,0) = \partial_t U_y(x,0) = 0 \quad \text{for } x \neq y\ .$$

Consider the wave equation in the whole three-dimensional space with appropriate initial conditions:

$$\begin{cases} \partial_t^2 u - \nabla \cdot \left(\chi(\mathbb{R}^3 \setminus \overline{D}) + k\chi(D) \right)\nabla u = \delta_{x=y}\delta_{t=0} \quad \text{in } \mathbb{R}^3 \times]0, +\infty[\ , \\ u(x,0) = 0, \quad \partial_t u(x,0) = 0 \quad \text{for } x \in \mathbb{R}^3, x \neq y\ . \end{cases} \tag{8.9}$$

Let $\delta u := u - U$ denote the perturbation due to the anomaly. Set $T = |y-z|$. Note that $U_y(z,t) \neq 0$ if and only if $t = T$. Using the method of matched asymptotic expansions, we can find that, for $x \in D$ and $t = t(x) \approx T$,

$$u(x,t) \approx U(z,T) + \delta\hat{v}_1(\frac{x-z}{\delta}) \cdot \nabla U_y(z,T)\ , \tag{8.10}$$

where $\hat{v}_1$ is given by (7.4). Hence, by (8.10) $\Delta u \approx 0$ in D. It then follows that

$$\left(\partial_t^2 - \Delta\right)\delta u = \left(\left.\frac{\partial u}{\partial \nu}\right|_+ - \left.\frac{\partial u}{\partial \nu}\right|_-\right)\delta_{\partial D} + (k-1)\chi(D)\Delta u \approx (1 - \frac{1}{k})\left.\frac{\partial u}{\partial \nu}\right|_+ \delta_{\partial D} ,$$

where $\delta_{\partial D}$ is the surface Dirac function on ∂D. Therefore, by once again (8.10) together with an integral representation formula for δu, we can readily get

$$\delta u(x,t) \approx (\frac{1}{k} - 1)\int_0^t \int_{\partial D} \frac{\delta_{\tau=t-|x-x'|}}{4\pi|x-x'|}\left.\frac{\partial u}{\partial \nu}\right|_+ (x',\tau)\, d\sigma(x')\, d\tau ,$$

and thus,

$$\delta u(x,t) \approx (\frac{1}{k} - 1)\int_{\partial D} \frac{\delta_{t=|x-x'|+T}}{4\pi|x-x'|}\left.\frac{\partial \hat{v}_1}{\partial \nu}\right|_+ (\frac{x'-z}{\delta})\, d\sigma(x') \cdot \nabla U_y(z,T) .$$

The jump condition on the normal derivative of $\hat{v}_1$ yields

$$\delta u(x,t) \approx -(k-1)\int_{\partial D} \frac{\delta_{t=|x-x'|+T}}{4\pi|x-x'|}\left.\frac{\partial \hat{v}_1}{\partial \nu}\right|_- (\frac{x'-z}{\delta})\, d\sigma(x') \cdot \nabla U_y(z,T) .$$

Now for $|x-z| \gg \delta$, it follows from the identity

$$(k-1)\int_{\partial B} \xi \left.\frac{\partial \hat{v}_1}{\partial \nu}\right|_- (\xi)\, d\sigma(\xi) = M(k,B) ,$$

that

$$\delta u(x,t) \approx -\delta^3 \nabla(\frac{\delta_{t=|x-x'|-T}}{4\pi|x-x'|})\Big|_{x'=z} M(k,B)\nabla U_y(z,T) ,$$

or equivalently,

$$\delta u(x,t) \approx -\delta^3 \nabla U_z(x,t-T)M(k,B)\nabla U_y(z,T), \quad t > T .$$

Theorem 8.3.2 (Pointwise Perturbations) *Let u be the solution to (8.9). Set U_y to be the background solution. The following expansion holds*

$$(u - U_y)(x,t) \approx -\delta^3 \nabla U_z(x,t-T)M(k,B)\nabla U_y(z,T) \quad for\ t > T , \quad (8.11)$$

for x away from z, where $T = |y - z|$, $M(k,B)$ is defined by (7.3), and U_y and U_z are given by (8.8).

Theorem 8.3.2 says that the perturbation due to the anomaly is a wave emitted from the point z at $t = T$. The anomaly behaves like a dipolar source. Moreover, by the symmetry of the polarization tensor, (8.11) satisfies a reciprocity principle, the statement of which is that the perturbation measured at the source location is the same when one interchanges the source and anomaly locations. We should be careful with the interpretation of Formula (8.11). As shown in [6], (8.11) is valid only after truncating the high-frequency components (for frequencies $\omega \gg O(\delta^{-\alpha})$ for some $\alpha < 1/2$) of u, U_y, and U_z.

Time-Reversal Technique

To image the anomaly by a time-reversal technique, one measures the perturbation on a closed surface surrounding the anomaly, and retransmits it through the background medium in a time-reversed chronology. Then the perturbation will travel back to the location of the anomaly.

More precisely, let $p = M(k, B)\nabla U_y(z, T)$. By changing the origin of time, T can be set to 0 without loss of generality.

Suppose now that we are able to measure the perturbation $u - U$ and its normal derivative at any point x on a sphere S englobing the anomaly D during the interval $[0, t_0]$ for t_0 large enough. The time-reversal operation is described by the transform $t \mapsto t_0 - t$. Both the perturbation $u - U$ and its normal derivative on S are time-reversed and emitted from S. Then a time-reversed perturbation, denoted by $(u - U)_{\mathrm{tr}}$, propagates inside the volume Ω surrounded by S.

Taking into account the definition (8.8) of the outgoing fundamental solution, spatial reciprocity and time reversal invariance of the wave equation, it can be shown from Theorem 8.3.2 that the following expression for the time-reversed perturbation $(u - U)_{\mathrm{tr}}$ due to the anomaly D holds in Ω:

$$(u - U)_{\mathrm{tr}}(x, t) \approx -\delta^3 p \cdot \int_{\mathbb{R}} \int_S \left[U_x(x', t - \tau) \frac{\partial \nabla_z U_z}{\partial \nu}(x', t_0 - \tau) \right.$$
$$\left. - \nabla_z U_z(x', t_0 - \tau) \frac{\partial U_x}{\partial \nu}(x', t - \tau) \right] d\sigma(x') \, d\tau \ ,$$

$$\approx -\delta^3 p \cdot \nabla_z \int_{\mathbb{R}} \int_S \left[U_x(x', t - \tau) \frac{\partial U_z}{\partial \nu}(x', t_0 - \tau) \right.$$
$$\left. - U_z(x', t_0 - \tau) \frac{\partial U_x}{\partial \nu}(x', t - \tau) \right] d\sigma(x') \, d\tau \ ,$$

where

$$U_x(x', t - \tau) = \frac{\delta_{t - \tau = |x - x'|}}{4\pi |x - x'|} \ .$$

Multiplying the equation

$$\left(\partial_\tau^2 - \Delta_{x'} \right) U_x(x', t - \tau) = \delta_{\tau = t} \delta_{x' = x} \ ,$$

by $U_z(x', t_0 - \tau)$, integrating by parts, and using the equation

$$\left(\partial_\tau^2 - \Delta_{x'} \right) U_z(x', t_0 - \tau) = \delta_{\tau = t_0} \delta_{x' = z} \ ,$$

we have

$$\int_{\mathbb{R}} \int_S \left[U_x(x', t - \tau) \frac{\partial U_z}{\partial \nu}(x', t_0 - \tau) - U_z(x', t_0 - \tau) \frac{\partial U_x}{\partial \nu}(x', t - \tau) \right] d\sigma(x') \, d\tau$$
$$= U_z(x, t_0 - t) - U_z(x, t - t_0) \ ,$$

$$(8.12)$$

and therefore,

$$(u - U)_{\mathrm{tr}}(x, t) \approx -\delta^3 p \cdot \nabla \left(U_z(x, t_0 - t) - U_z(x, t - t_0) \right) . \qquad (8.13)$$

Equation (8.13) can be interpreted as the superposition of incoming and outgoing spherical waves, centered on the location z of the anomaly. Note that $(u - U)_{\mathrm{tr}}$ remains finite for all time although the incoming and outgoing spherical waves show a singularity at the point z.

By taking Fourier transform of (8.13) over the time variable t, we obtain that

$$\mathcal{F}((u - U)_{\mathrm{tr}})(x, \omega) \propto \delta^3 p \cdot \nabla \left(\frac{\sin(\omega |x - z|)}{|x - z|} \right) ,$$

where ω is the wavenumber. This shows that the time-reversal perturbation $(u - U)_{\mathrm{tr}}$ focuses on the location z of the anomaly with a focal spot size limited to one-half the wavelength which is in agreement with the Rayleigh resolution limit. It should be pointed out that in the frequency domain, (8.13) is only valid for $2\pi/\omega \gg \delta$.

Connection with the Helmholtz Equation, the MUSIC-type Algorithm and Backpropagation

Taking the Fourier transform of (8.9) over the time variable t yields the Helmholtz equation:

$$\nabla \cdot \left(\chi(\mathbb{R}^3 \setminus \overline{D}) + k\chi(D) \right) \nabla \hat{u} + \omega^2 \hat{u} = -\delta_{x=y} \quad \text{in} \quad \mathbb{R}^3 ,$$

where $\omega > 0$. Place on $\hat{u}$ the outgoing radiation condition. The background solution is $\widehat{U}_y(x, \omega) = e^{i\omega|x-y|}/(4\pi|x-y|)$. As $\delta \to 0$, the following asymptotic expansion for the perturbation $\delta \hat{u}$ due to the anomaly holds:

$$\delta \hat{u}(x, \omega) \approx \delta^3 \nabla \widehat{U}_z(x, \omega) M(k, B) \nabla \widehat{U}_y(z, \omega) \qquad (8.14)$$

for x away from z, where $\widehat{U}_z(x, \omega) = e^{i\omega|x-z|}/(4\pi|x - z|)$.

Suppose that one measures the perturbation $\delta \hat{u}$ and its normal derivative on a sphere S englobing the anomaly D. To detect the anomaly D one computes

$$\hat{w}(x, \omega) := \int_S \left[\widehat{U}_x(x', \omega) \overline{\frac{\partial \delta \hat{u}}{\partial \nu}}(x', \omega) - \overline{\delta \hat{u}(x', \omega)} \frac{\partial \widehat{U}_x}{\partial \nu}(x', \omega) \right] d\sigma(x') ,$$

in the domain Ω surrounded by S. Observe that $\hat{w}(x, \omega)$ is a solution to the Helmholtz equation: $(\Delta + \omega^2)\hat{w} = 0$ in Ω.

The following identity, parallel to (8.12), plays a key role in achieving the resolution limit. Applying Green's theorem to $\widehat{U}_x(x', \omega)$ and $\overline{\widehat{U}_z(x', \omega)}$, we have

$$\int_S \left[\widehat{U}_x(x',\omega) \overline{\frac{\partial \widehat{U}_z}{\partial \nu}(x',\omega)} - \widehat{U}_z(x',\omega) \overline{\frac{\partial \widehat{U}_x}{\partial \nu}(x',\omega)} \right] d\sigma(x') = -2i\Im m\, \widehat{U}_z(x,\omega)\,.$$

$$(8.15)$$

In view of (8.15), we immediately find from the asymptotic expansion (8.14) that

$$\hat{w}(x,\omega) \propto \delta^3 \hat{p} \cdot \nabla \left(\frac{\sin(\omega|x-z|)}{|x-z|} \right)\,, \qquad (8.16)$$

where $\hat{p} = M(k,B)\nabla \widehat{U}_y(z,\omega)$, which shows that $\hat{w}(x,\omega)$ has a peak at the location z of the anomaly and also proves the Rayleigh resolution limit.

A formula similar to (8.16) can be derived in an inhomogeneous medium Ω surrounded by S. If $\hat{w}(x,\omega)$ denotes the solution computed from $\delta \hat{u}$ and its normal derivative on S by

$$\hat{w}(x,\omega) = \int_S \left[G(x,x',\omega) \overline{\frac{\partial \delta \hat{u}}{\partial \nu}(x',\omega)} - \overline{\delta \hat{u}(x',\omega)} \frac{\partial G}{\partial \nu}(x,x',\omega) \right] d\sigma(x')\,,$$

where G is the Green function in the inhomogeneous medium Ω, then we have

$$\hat{w}(x,\omega) \propto \nabla \Im m\, G(x,z,\omega)\,,$$

which shows that the sharper the behavior of $\Im m\, G$ at z, the higher the resolution.

We now turn to the connection with the backpropagation- and MUSIC-type algorithms. Let $(y_1,\dots,y_n)$ be n (equidistant) points on S. The MUSIC-type algorithm for locating D reads:

$$x \approx z \quad \text{if and only if} \quad \frac{1}{\left| \dfrac{\omega^2}{16\pi^2 R^2} - \dfrac{1}{n}\displaystyle\sum_{l=1}^n \nabla \widehat{U}_{y_l}(x,\omega) \cdot \overline{\nabla \widehat{U}_z(y_l,\omega)} \right|} \approx +\infty\,,$$

$$(8.17)$$

as the radius R of the sphere S goes to $+\infty$ while the backpropagation-type algorithm is as follows:

$$x \approx z \quad \text{if and only if} \quad \frac{1}{n}\sum_{l=1}^n \nabla \widehat{U}_{y_l}(x,\omega) \cdot \overline{\nabla \widehat{U}_z(y_l,\omega)} \approx \frac{\omega^2}{16\pi^2 R^2}\,.$$

For sufficiently large n, we have

$$\frac{1}{n}\sum_{l=1}^n \nabla \widehat{U}_{y_l}(x,\omega) \cdot \overline{\nabla \widehat{U}_z(y_l,\omega)} \approx \frac{1}{4\pi R^2}\int_S \nabla \widehat{U}_y(x,\omega) \cdot \overline{\nabla \widehat{U}_z(y,\omega)}\, d\sigma(y)\,.$$

Since

$$4\pi \nabla_x \widehat{U}_y(x,\omega) = -i\omega \frac{e^{i\omega|y|}}{|y|}\frac{y}{|y|}e^{-i\omega \frac{y}{|y|}\cdot x} + O(\frac{1}{|y|^2})\,,$$

it follows that

$$\int_S \nabla \widehat{U}_y(x,\omega) \cdot \overline{\nabla \widehat{U}_z(y,\omega)} \, d\sigma(y) \approx \frac{\omega^2}{16\pi^2 R^2} \int_S e^{-i\omega \frac{y}{|y|} \cdot (z-x)} \, d\sigma(y) = \frac{\omega^2}{4\pi} j_0(\omega|z-x|),$$

as $R \to +\infty$, where j_0 is the spherical Bessel function of order zero. Hence,

$$\frac{1}{n} \sum_{l=1}^{n} \nabla \widehat{U}_{y_l}(x,\omega) \cdot \overline{\nabla \widehat{U}_z(y_l,\omega)} \approx \frac{\omega^2}{16\pi^2 R^2} j_0(\omega|z-x|) \quad \left(\propto \Im m \, \widehat{U}_z(x,\omega) \right),$$

which, if one compares with (8.16), shows that time-reversal and backpropagation have the same resolution while (8.17) reduces to the following

$$x \approx z \quad \text{if and only if} \quad \frac{6R^2}{16\pi^2 \omega^4 |z - x|^2} \approx +\infty \, ;$$

and so clearly proves that the MUSIC-type algorithm achieves a sub-wavelength detection.

Bibliography and Discussion

The anomaly detection techniques developed in this chapter could be seen as a regularizing method in comparison with iterative approaches; they reduce the set of admissible solution. Their robustness is related to the fact that the number of unknowns is reduced.

The projection algorithm was introduced in [87, 20]. The MUSIC algorithm was originally developed for source separation in signal theory [119]. The MUSIC-type algorithm for locating small electromagnetic anomalies from the multi-static response matrix at a fixed frequency was developed in [9]. A variety of numerical results was presented in [9, 10, 11] to highlight its potential and their limitation.

In the case where the data is a discrete version of the Neumann-to-Dirichlet boundary map, Brühl, Hanke, and Vogelius [32] were the first to use the asymptotic perturbation formula (7.2) for small conductivity anomalies in combination with MUSIC ideas to design a very effective algorithm to determine the locations of the anomalies. The Neumann functions at the locations of the anomalies are the eigenvalues of the leading-order term in the asymptotic expansion of the perturbations in the Neumann-to-Dirichlet boundary map that are due to the presence of the anomalies. Naturally, and in accordance with the results proven in [62] on the optimal current pattern problem, these functions are the optimal currents to apply in order to image the anomalies.

Theorem 8.3.1 is from [3] and Theorem 8.3.2 is from [6]. The inverse problems of identifying locations and certain properties of the shapes of small anomalies from dynamic boundary measurements on only part of the boundary and for a finite interval in time have been considered in [3]. In that paper, a non-iterative algorithm for solving the inverse problems has been proposed using as weights particular background solutions constructed by a geometrical control method. See [15] for the reconstruction of elastic anomalies in the time-domain.

The physical literature on time-reversal is quite rich. See [56] and the references therein. Some interesting mathematical works started to deal with different aspects of time-reversal phenomena: see, for instance, [26] for time-reversal in the time-domain, [50, 97, 64, 37, 38] for time-reversal in the frequency domain, and [60, 29] for time-reversal in random media.

Up to now, the main clinical application of time-reversal is in ultrasound therapy (tumor or kidney stone destruction). But, as shown in Sect. 8.3, time-reversal is expected to lead to a very effective method for anomaly detection. Focusing on the anomaly may be achieved without any knowledge of the background medium. When a medium contains several anomalies, after a first illumination of the medium, the reflected wavefronts can be recorded and time-reversed. This process can be repeated iteratively. It has been shown by Prada and Fink in [109] that this process converges and produces a wavefront focused on the most conductive anomaly. See also [110]. The theoretical analysis of this iterative time-reversal process led to an elegant method, known as the DORT method (decomposition of the time-reversal operator in French).

It is worth mentioning that the MUSIC-type algorithm developed in this chapter is related to the linear sampling method of Colton and Kirsch [43]. We refer to Cheney [39], Kirsch [83], and the recent paper [7] for detailed discussions of the connection between MUSIC-type algorithms and the linear sampling method. Our MUSIC algorithm is also related to time-reversal [110, 97]. With the notation of Sect. 8.2, if A is the multi-static response matrix then $\bar{A}$ is the frequency-domain version of a time-reversed multi-static response matrix. Thus the matrix $\tilde{A} = \bar{A}A$ corresponds to performing an experiment, time-reversed the received signals and using them as input for a second experiment. The backpropagation algorithm briefly described in the last section is the analogous of the time-reversal in the frequency domain. The DORT method is nothing else than saying that the corresponding eigenvectors of $\bar{A}A$ generate incident waves that focus selectively on the anomalies. As shown in [9], this result is not true in general, but does hold for small and well-separated anomalies with distinct electromagnetic parameters. See also [64] for point-like (or purely dielectric) anomalies. The MUSIC algorithm could be seen as a post-processor to the DORT approach.

The MUSIC algorithm can be adapted to MEG/EEG source localization. Recursively applied and projected MUSIC (RAP-MUSIC) is a recent extension of MUSIC for MEG and EEG applications. RAP-MUSIC refines the MUSIC cost function after each source is found by projecting the signal subspace away from the singular vectors corresponding to the sources already found. See [23].

Finally, it is worth emphasizing that the methods presented in this chapter enable to detect the locations and the PT from the boundary measurements. It is the detected PT which yields an information about the size (and orientation) of the anomaly. However, the information from the PT is a mixture of the conductivity and the volume. It is impossible to extract the conductivity from the PT. A small anomaly with high conductivity and larger anomaly with lower conductivity can have the same PT. It would be interesting and important to extract information about the property of the anomaly from boundary measurements. It is likely that internal measurements yield such information.

Part IV

Hybrid Imaging Techniques

9

Magnetic Resonance Electrical Impedance Tomography

Magnetic resonance electrical impedance tomography (MREIT) is an imaging technique of reconstructing the cross-sectional conductivity distribution of a human body by means of the EIT technique integrated with the MRI technique.

In MREIT, one uses a magnetic resonance imaging scanner to measure the induced magnetic flux density due to an injection current. When one injects a current into a subject, it produces a magnetic field as well as an electric field. In EIT, one utilizes only the electrical quantities. Furthermore, since there is no noninvasive way of getting measurements of electrical quantities from inside the subject, we are limited in EIT by the boundary current-voltage data which is insensitive to internal conductivity perturbations. However, one can enrich the data by measuring the internal magnetic flux density. This can be done using a magnetic resonance imaging scanner as a tool to capture the internal magnetic flux density images. This technique is called magnetic resonance current density imaging (MRCDI). Combining EIT and MRCDI, MREIT perceives the distortion of current pathways due to the conductivity distribution to be imaged and overcomes the severe ill-posedness character of EIT.

In this chapter, we first formulate the forward and inverse problem in MREIT utilizing the internal magnetic flux density in conductivity image reconstructions. Then we discuss the uniqueness issue in MREIT. We show that one should use at least two appropriate injection currents for the uniqueness of reconstructed conductivity image. After that, we describe the J-substitution algorithm which provides a high-resolution conductivity image. This algorithm is involved with a nonlinear partial differential equation instead of the linear conductivity equation.

9.1 Mathematical Model

Let us explain the mathematical model in MREIT. Let the body occupy a bounded domain $\Omega \subset \mathbb{R}^d, d = 2, 3$. When a current density $g \in L_0^2(\partial\Omega)$ is injected through the outer surface of the body Ω, it induces an electrical potential distribution u that satisfies the two-dimensional conductivity equation

$$\begin{cases} \nabla_x \cdot (\gamma(x)\nabla_x u) = 0 \text{ in } \Omega , \\[2mm] \gamma(x)\dfrac{\partial u}{\partial \nu} = g \text{ on } \partial\Omega , \\[2mm] \displaystyle\int_{\partial\Omega} u = 0 , \end{cases} \qquad (9.1)$$

where $\gamma(x)$ denotes the conductivity coefficient of the body which we want to reconstruct. The function γ may be regarded as a piecewise continuous function because distinct tissues have different conductivities.

With this current g, the resulting internal current density vector is

$$\mathbf{J} = -\gamma\nabla u .$$

The presence of the internal current density $\mathbf{J}$ generates a magnetic flux density $\mathbf{B}$ and Ampére's law $\mathbf{J} = (1/\mu_0) \nabla \times \mathbf{B}$ holds inside the electrically conducting subject, where the constant μ_0 is the magnetic permeability of Ω. Suppose $d = 3$ and let the x_3-axis be the direction of the main magnetic field of the MRI scanner. Using the MRI scanner, we can measure B_3, the third component of $\mathbf{B}$. According to the Biot-Savart law, B_3 can be expressed as

$$B_3(x) = \frac{\mu_0}{4\pi} \int_\Omega \frac{\gamma(x')}{|x - x'|^3} \left[(x_1 - x_1')\partial_2 u(x') - (x_2 - x_2')\partial_1 u(x') \right] dx' \qquad (9.2)$$

for $x = (x_1, x_2, x_3) \in \Omega$.

Assuming that one can rotate the subject, the MREIT system furnishes the internal data $J := |\mathbf{J}| = \gamma|\nabla u|$, which is measured and processed in the MRI system.

Substituting

$$\gamma(x) = \frac{J(x)}{|\nabla u(x)|}, \quad x \in \Omega ,$$

into the conductivity equation (9.1), we obtain that u satisfies the following nonlinear Neumann boundary value problem (the 1–Laplacian)

$$\begin{cases} \nabla \cdot \left(\dfrac{J}{|\nabla u|}\nabla u \right) = 0 \text{ in } \Omega , \\[3mm] \dfrac{J}{|\nabla u|}\dfrac{\partial u}{\partial \nu} = g \text{ on } \partial\Omega , \\[3mm] \displaystyle\int_{\partial\Omega} u = 0 . \end{cases} \qquad (9.3)$$

Unfortunately, once (9.3) has a solution, then it always has infinitely many solutions. Consequently, the model may have infinitely many distinct conductivity images. Moreover, (9.3) in general does not have an existence result even if γ is smooth. Thus the model is not appropriate for making a reconstruction algorithm and should be modified in order to guarantee the uniqueness. This can be done by using two current patterns g_1, and g_2, and imposing that

$$\gamma = \frac{J_1}{|\nabla u_1|} = \frac{J_2}{|\nabla u_2|} \in \Sigma,$$

Σ being the class of piecewise continuous functions. Doing so, we arrive at the following nonlinear system:

$$\begin{cases} \nabla_x \cdot \left(\dfrac{J_i(x)}{|\nabla u_i|} \nabla u_i \right) = 0 \ \text{ in } \Omega, \\[2mm] \dfrac{J_i(x)}{|\nabla u_i|} \dfrac{\partial u_i}{\partial \nu} = g_i \text{ on } \partial\Omega, \\[2mm] \dfrac{J_1}{|\nabla u_1|} = \dfrac{J_2}{|\nabla u_2|} \in \Sigma, \\[2mm] \displaystyle\int_{\partial\Omega} u_i = 0. \end{cases} \tag{9.4}$$

For the uniqueness of a solution to the nonlinear system (9.4), the appropriate pair of current patterns g_1 and g_2 has to be chosen such that

$$|\nabla u_1(x) \times \nabla u_2(x)| > 0 \quad \text{for all } x \in \Omega.$$

The following result is of importance to us.

Lemma 9.1.1 *Suppose $d = 2$. Suppose that g is such that there exist two disjoint arcs $\partial\Omega^+$ and $\partial\Omega^-$ contained in $\partial\Omega$ such that*

$$\partial\Omega^+ \cup \partial\Omega^- = \partial\Omega \quad \text{and} \quad \partial\Omega^+ \subset \{g \geq 0\}, \quad \partial\Omega^- \subset \{g \leq 0\}. \tag{9.5}$$

Let u be the solution to (9.1). Then $\nabla u(x) \neq 0$ for all $x \in \Omega$.

In practice, the current is applied through pairs of electrodes attached at points on the boundary $\partial\Omega$. Here, let P_1, P_2, Q_1, and Q_2 be situated along $\partial\Omega$ in this order and separated by a distance greater than 2δ. Suppose that

$$g_j(x) = \begin{cases} +\frac{I}{2\delta} & \text{on } \{|x - P_j| < \delta\} \cap \partial\Omega, \\[2mm] -\frac{I}{2\delta} & \text{on } \{|x - Q_j| < \delta\} \cap \partial\Omega, \\[2mm] 0 & \text{otherwise,} \end{cases} \tag{9.6}$$

where I is the current sent to both electrodes P_j and Q_j, and 2δ is the width of each electrode. With these currents, we can easily see that the solution (u_1, u_2) to (9.4) satisfies $\nabla u_j(x) \neq 0$ for all $x \in \Omega, j = 1, 2$.

Moreover, using Lemma 9.1.1, we obtain the following.

Lemma 9.1.2 *Suppose $d = 2$. Suppose that (u_1, u_2) is a solution to the non-linear system (9.4) with the Neumann data g_1 and g_2 defined in (9.6). Then we have*

$$|\nabla u_1(x) \times \nabla u_2(x)| > 0 \quad \text{for all } x \in \Omega .$$

Lemma 9.1.2 tells us that ∇u_1 and ∇u_2 are neither vanishing nor parallel to each other at any points in Ω. Based on this fact, one can prove that the region where the conductivity distribution has jumps can be uniquely detected by the observation of the discontinuities of the measured data (J_1, J_2).

Theorem 9.1.3 (Edge Detection) *Suppose $d = 2$. Suppose that (u_1, u_2), $(\tilde{u}_1, \tilde{u}_2)$ are solutions to the nonlinear system (9.4) with the Neumann data g_1 and g_2 defined in (9.6). Then the edge of the conductivity image is uniquely determined by (J_1, J_2) in such a way that*

$$\left\{ x : \frac{J_i}{|\nabla u_i|} \text{ is discontinuous at } x \right\} = \left\{ x : \frac{J_i}{|\nabla \tilde{u}_i|} \text{ is discontinuous at } x \right\} .$$

When the conductivity distribution is known to be piecewise constant, one can show that the edge of the conductivity image as well as the conductivity values can be determined.

Theorem 9.1.4 (Uniqueness) *Suppose $d = 2$. Suppose that (u_1, u_2), $(\tilde{u}_1, \tilde{u}_2)$ are solutions to the nonlinear system (9.4) with the Neumann data g_1 and g_2 defined in (9.6). Suppose that $J_i/|\nabla u_i|$ and $J_i/|\nabla \tilde{u}_i|$ are piecewise constants. Then (u_1, u_2) and $(\tilde{u}_1, \tilde{u}_2)$ are the same.*

9.2 J-Substitution Algorithm

The J-substitution algorithm uses two injection currents satisfying (9.6) and is based on an iterative scheme of the following coupled system:

$$\begin{cases} \nabla_x \cdot \left(\dfrac{J_i(x)}{|\nabla u_i|} \nabla u_i \right) = 0 \ \text{ in } \Omega , \quad (i = 1, 2) \\[2mm] \dfrac{J_1(x)}{|\nabla u_1|} = \dfrac{J_2(x)}{|\nabla u_2|} \ \text{ in } \Omega , \\[2mm] \dfrac{J_i(x)}{|\nabla u_i|} \dfrac{\partial u_i}{\partial \nu} = g_i \ \text{ on } \partial\Omega , \\[2mm] \displaystyle\int_{\partial\Omega} u_i = 0 . \end{cases} \tag{9.7}$$

The following is the J-substitution algorithm:

(i) Initial guess $\gamma_0 = 1$.
(ii) For each $n = 0, 1, \ldots$, solve

$$\begin{cases} \nabla_x \cdot (\gamma_n(x) \nabla_x u_1^n) = 0 \text{ in } \Omega, \\[2mm] \gamma_n(x) \dfrac{\partial u_1^n}{\partial \nu} = g_1 \text{ on } \partial\Omega, \\[2mm] \displaystyle\int_{\partial\Omega} u_1^n = 0. \end{cases}$$

(iii) Update $\gamma_{n+1/2} \Leftarrow J_1/|\nabla u_1^n|$.
(iv) Solve

$$\begin{cases} \nabla_x \cdot \left(\gamma_{n+1/2}(x) \nabla_x u_2^{n+1/2}\right) = 0 \text{ in } \Omega , \\[2mm] \gamma_{n+1/2}(x) \dfrac{\partial u_2^{n+1/2}}{\partial \nu} = g_2 \text{ on } \partial\Omega , \\[2mm] \displaystyle\int_{\partial\Omega} u_2^{n+1/2} = 0 . \end{cases}$$

(v) Update $\gamma_{n+1} \Leftarrow J_2/|\nabla u_2^{n+1/2}|$.
(vi) Repeat the process (ii)-(iv) until $\left| J_2 - \gamma_{n+1}|\nabla u_2^n| \right| < \epsilon$.

The J-substitution algorithm has been successfully demonstrated to provide accurate high-resolution conductivity images. See Fig. 9.1.

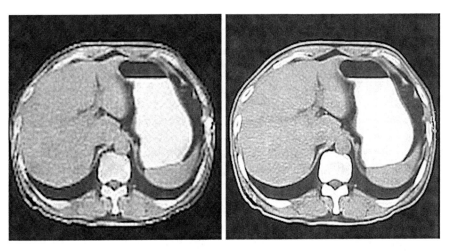

Fig. 9.1. J-substitution algorithm: a simulation by O. Kwon, E. Woo, J. Yoon, and J.K. Seo.

9.3 The Harmonic Algorithm

The J-substitution algorithm suffers from the subject rotation process. In order to eliminate this subject rotation, we should solve the problem of reconstructing γ from only B_3 data instead of complete set of data for $\mathbf{B}$.

As in J-substitution algorithm, we apply two currents g_1 and g_2 through electrodes placed on $\partial\Omega$ and measure the third components of the induced magnetic flux densities, B_3^1 and B_3^2. The harmonic algorithm is based on the following identity derived from Ampére's law:

$$
\begin{bmatrix} \dfrac{\partial\gamma}{\partial x} \\[2mm] \dfrac{\partial\gamma}{\partial y} \end{bmatrix} = \frac{1}{\mu_0} \begin{bmatrix} \dfrac{\partial u_1[\gamma]}{\partial y} & -\dfrac{\partial u_1[\gamma]}{\partial x} \\[3mm] \dfrac{\partial u_2[\gamma]}{\partial y} & -\dfrac{\partial u_2[\gamma]}{\partial x} \end{bmatrix}^{-1} \begin{bmatrix} \Delta B_3^1 \\[1mm] \Delta B_3^2 \end{bmatrix}, \tag{9.8}
$$

where $u_j[\gamma]$ is the solution of (9.1).

Using the identity (9.8), we have the following representation formula for each slice $\Omega \cap \{x_3 = a\}$:

$$
\begin{aligned}
\gamma(x_1, x_2, a) &= H_\gamma(x_1, x_2, a) \\
&- \int_{\Omega\cap\{x_3=a\}} \frac{(x_1 - x_1' \, , \, x_2 - x_2')}{\sqrt{|x_1 - x_1'|^2 + |x_2 - x_2'|^2}} \cdot \mathbb{A}^{-1}[\gamma] \begin{bmatrix} \Delta B_3^1 \\ \Delta B_3^2 \end{bmatrix} dx_1' dx_2'
\end{aligned} \tag{9.9}
$$

where

$$
\mathbb{A}[\gamma] := 2\pi\mu_0 \begin{bmatrix} \partial_2 u_1[\gamma] & -\partial_1 u_1[\gamma] \\ \partial_2 u_2[\gamma] & -\partial_1 u_2[\gamma] \end{bmatrix} \tag{9.10}
$$

and

$$
H_\gamma(x_1, x_2, a) := \int_{\partial(\Omega\cap\{x_3=a\})} \frac{(x_1 - x_1' \, , \, x_2 - x_2') \cdot \nu}{2\pi\sqrt{|x_1 - x_1'|^2 + |x_2 - x_2'|^2}} \gamma(x_1', x_2', a) \, d\sigma' \, .
$$

Here, ν is the two dimensional unit outward normal vector to the boundary $\partial(\Omega \cap \{x_3 = a\})$ and $d\sigma'$ is the line element. Note that H_γ is harmonic in the two-dimensional slice $\Omega\cap\{x_3 = a\}$. It is known if γ is known on the boundary $\partial(\Omega \cap \{x_3 = a\})$.

The harmonic algorithm for reconstructing γ is a natural iterative procedure of the identity (9.9). Suppose for simplicity that γ is known on the boundary, say $\gamma \equiv 1$ on $\partial(\Omega \cap \{x_3 = a\})$. The Harmonic algorithm is as follows:

(i) Let $n = 0$. Solve (9.1) for u_j^0 with $\gamma = 1$ and $g = g_j$.
(ii) Compute γ_{n+1} using (9.9) with u_j replacing u_j^n.
(iii) Compute $u_j^{n+1}, j = 1, 2$, by solving (9.1) with $\gamma = \gamma_{n+1}$.
(iv) If $\|\gamma_{n+1} - \gamma_n\|_2 < \epsilon$, stop and set $\gamma = \gamma_{n+1}$. Here, ϵ is a given tolerance. Otherwise, set $n \leftarrow (n + 1)$ and go to Step (ii).

Bibliography and Discussion

This chapter was devoted to the breakthrough work by J.K. Seo and his group. The results of this chapter are from [81, 88, 80]. A rigorous convergence analysis of the J-substitution algorithm is still missing. Very recently, some progress on the convergence and the stability of the harmonic algorithm has been made in [93].

10

Impediography

Impediography is another mathematical direction for future EIT research in view of biomedical applications. It keeps the most important merits of EIT (real time imaging, low cost, portability). It is based on the simultaneous measurement of an electric current and of acoustic vibrations induced by ultrasound waves. Its intrinsic resolution depends on the size of the focal spot of the acoustic perturbation, and thus it provides high resolution images.

The core idea of impediography is to extract more information about the conductivity from data that has been enriched by coupling the electric measurements to localized elastic perturbations. More precisely, one perturbs the medium during the electric measurements, by focusing ultrasonic waves on regions of small diameter inside the body. Using a simple model for the mechanical effects of the ultrasound waves, we can show that the difference between the measurements in the unperturbed and perturbed configurations is asymptotically equal to the pointwise value of the energy density at the center of the perturbed zone. In practice, the ultrasounds impact a zone of a few millimeters in diameter. The perturbation should thus be sensitive to conductivity variations at the millimeter scale, which is the precision required for breast cancer diagnostic.

10.1 Physical Model

A body (a domain $\Omega \subset \mathbb{R}^2$) is electrically probed: One or several currents are imposed on the surface and the induced potentials are measured on the boundary. At the same time, a circular region of a few millimeters in the interior of Ω is mechanically excited by ultrasonic waves, which dilate this region. The measurements are made as the focus of the ultrasounds scans the entire domain. Several sets of measurements can be obtained by varying the ultrasound waves amplitudes and the applied currents.

Within each (small) disk volume, the conductivity is assumed to be constant per volume unit. At a point $x \in \Omega$, within a disk B of volume V_B, the electric conductivity γ is defined in terms of a density ρ as $\gamma(x) = \rho(x)V_B$.

The ultrasonic waves induce a small elastic deformation of the sphere B. See Fig. 10.1. If this deformation is isotropic, the material points of B occupy a volume V_B^p in the perturbed configuration, which at first order is equal to

$$V_B^p = V_B(1 + 2\frac{\Delta r}{r}) ,$$

where r is the radius of the disk B and Δr is the variation of the radius due to the elastic perturbation. As Δr is proportional to the amplitude of the ultrasonic wave, we obtain a proportional change of the deformation. Using two different ultrasonic waves with different amplitudes but with the same spot, it is therefore easy to compute the ratio V_B^p/V_B. As a consequence, the perturbed electrical conductivity γ^p satisfies

$$\forall\, x \in \Omega, \quad \gamma^p(x) = \rho(x)V_B^p \;=\; \gamma(x)\nu(x) ,$$

where $\nu(x) = V_B^p/V_B$ is a known function. We make the following realistic assumptions: (i) the ultrasonic wave expands the zone it impacts, and changes its conductivity: $\forall x \in \Omega$, $\nu(x) > 1$, and (ii) the perturbation is not too small: $\nu(x) - 1 \gg V_B$.

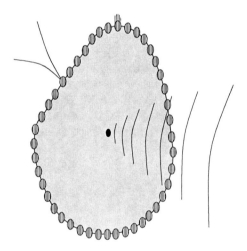

Fig. 10.1. Experimental setup.

10.2 Mathematical Model

We denote by u the voltage potential induced by a current g, in the absence of ultrasonic perturbations. It is given by

$$\begin{cases} \nabla_x \cdot (\gamma(x)\nabla_x u) = 0 \text{ in } \Omega , \\ \gamma(x)\dfrac{\partial u}{\partial \nu} = g \text{ on } \partial\Omega , \end{cases} \qquad (10.1)$$

with the convention that $\int_{\partial\Omega} u = 0$. We suppose that the conductivity γ is known close to the boundary of the domain, so that ultrasonic probing is limited to interior points. We denote the corresponding open set Ω_1 .

We denote by $u_\delta(x)$, $x \in \Omega$, the voltage potential induced by a current g, in the presence of ultrasonic perturbations localized in a disk-shaped domain $D := z + \delta B$ of volume $|D| = O(\delta^2)$. The voltage potential u_δ is a solution to

$$\begin{cases} \nabla_x \cdot (\gamma_\delta(x)\nabla_x u_\delta(x)) = 0 \text{ in } \Omega , \\ \gamma(x)\dfrac{\partial u_\delta}{\partial \nu} = g \text{ on } \partial\Omega , \end{cases} \qquad (10.2)$$

with the notation

$$\gamma_\delta(x) = \gamma(x)\left[1 + \chi(D)(x)\left(\nu(x) - 1\right)\right] ,$$

where $\chi(D)$ is the characteristic function of the domain D.

As the zone deformed by the ultrasound wave is small, we can view it as a small volume perturbation of the background conductivity γ, and seek an asymptotic expansion of the boundary values of $u_\delta - u$. The method of small volume expansions shows that comparing u_δ and u on $\partial\Omega$ provides information about the conductivity. Indeed, we can prove that

$$\int_{\partial\Omega}(u_\delta - u)g\,d\sigma = \int_D \gamma(x)\frac{(\nu(x)-1)^2}{\nu(x)+1}\nabla u \cdot \nabla u\,dx + o(|D|)$$

$$= |\nabla u(z)|^2 \int_D \gamma(x)\frac{(\nu(x)-1)^2}{\nu(x)+1}\,dx + o(|D|) .$$

Therefore, we have

$$\gamma(z)\,|\nabla u(z)|^2 = \mathcal{E}(z) + o(1) , \qquad (10.3)$$

where the function $\mathcal{E}(z)$ is defined by

$$\mathcal{E}(z) = \left(\int_D \frac{(\nu(x)-1)^2}{\nu(x)+1}dx\right)^{-1}\int_{\partial\Omega}(u_\delta - u)g\,d\sigma . \qquad (10.4)$$

By scanning the interior of the body with ultrasound waves, given an applied current g, we then obtain data from which we can compute

$$\mathcal{E}(z) := \gamma(z)|\nabla u(z)|^2 ,$$

in an interior sub–region of Ω. The new inverse problem is now to reconstruct γ knowing $\mathcal{E}$.

10.3 E-Substitution Algorithm

The use of $\mathcal{E}$ leads us to transform (10.1), having two unknowns γ and u with highly nonlinear dependency on γ, into the following nonlinear PDE (the 0–Laplacian)

$$
\begin{cases}
\nabla_x \cdot \left(\dfrac{\mathcal{E}}{|\nabla u|^2} \nabla u \right) = 0 \text{ in } \Omega\,, \\[2ex]
\dfrac{\mathcal{E}}{|\nabla u|^2} \dfrac{\partial u}{\partial \nu} = g \text{ on } \partial\Omega\,.
\end{cases}
\tag{10.5}
$$

We emphasize that $\mathcal{E}$ is a known function, constructed from the measured data (10.4). Consequently, all the parameters entering in equation (10.5) are known. So, the ill-posed inverse problem of EIT model is converted into less complicated direct problem (10.5). The E-substitution algorithm uses two currents g_1 and g_2. We choose this pair of current patterns to have $\nabla u_1 \times \nabla u_2 \neq 0$ for all $x \in \Omega$, where $u_i, i = 1, 2$, is the solution to (10.1). See Lemma 9.1.2 for an evidence of the possibility of such a choice.

The E-substitution algorithm is in the spirit of Subsect 5.1.4. It is based on an approximation of a linearized version of problem (10.5).

Suppose that γ is a small perturbation of conductivity profile γ_0: $\gamma = \gamma_0 + \delta\gamma$. Let u_0 and $u = u_0 + \delta u$ denote the potentials corresponding to γ_0 and γ with the same Neumann boundary data g. It is easily seen that δu satisfies $\nabla \cdot (\gamma \nabla \delta u) = -\nabla \cdot (\delta\gamma \nabla u_0)$ in Ω with the homogeneous Dirichlet boundary condition. Moreover, from

$$
\mathcal{E} = (\gamma_0 + \delta\gamma)|\nabla(u_0 + \delta u)|^2 \approx \gamma_0 |\nabla u_0|^2 + \delta\gamma |\nabla u_0|^2 + 2\gamma_0 \nabla u_0 \cdot \nabla \delta u\,,
$$

after neglecting the terms $\delta\gamma \nabla u_0 \cdot \nabla \delta u$ and $\delta\gamma |\nabla \delta u|^2$, it follows that

$$
\delta\gamma \approx \frac{\mathcal{E}}{|\nabla u_0|^2} - \gamma_0 - 2\gamma_0 \frac{\nabla \delta u \cdot \nabla u_0}{|\nabla u_0|^2}\,.
$$

The following is the E-substitution algorithm. We start from an initial guess for the conductivity γ, and solve the corresponding Dirichlet conductivity problem

$$
\begin{cases}
\nabla \cdot (\gamma \nabla u_0) = 0 \text{ in } \Omega\,, \\
u_0 = \psi \text{ on } \partial\Omega\,.
\end{cases}
$$

The data ψ is the Dirichlet data measured as a response to the current g (say $g = g_1$) in absence of elastic deformation.

The discrepancy between the data and our guessed solution is

$$
\epsilon_0 := \frac{\mathcal{E}}{|\nabla u_0|^2} - \gamma\,.
\tag{10.6}
$$

We then introduce a corrector, δu, computed as the solution to

$$\begin{cases} \nabla \cdot (\gamma \nabla \delta u) = -\nabla \cdot (\varepsilon_0 \nabla u_0) & \text{in } \Omega , \\ \delta u = 0 & \text{on } \partial\Omega , \end{cases}$$

and update the conductivity

$$\gamma := \frac{\mathcal{E} - 2\gamma \nabla \delta u \cdot \nabla u_0}{|\nabla u_0|^2} .$$

We iteratively update the conductivity, alternating directions (*i.e.*, with $g = g_2$).

The efficiency of this approach have been tested on various problems and domains. We present here one such test. The domain Ω is a disk of radius 8 centered at the origin, which contains three anomalies, an ellipse, an L-shaped domain and a triangle, so as to image a convex object, a non-convex object, and an object with a smooth boundary.

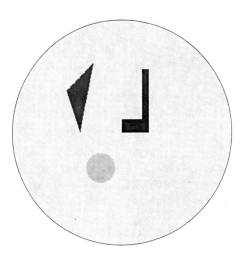

Fig. 10.2. Conductivity distribution.

The background conductivity is equal to 0.5, the conductivity takes the values 2 in the triangle, 0.75 in the ellipse and 2.55 in the L–shaped domain. See Fig. 10.2. We chose values corresponding to small and large contrast with the background. Note that the smaller the contrast the easier the detection. The choice of a significant contrast was not made to highlight the objects, but rather to make the reconstruction more challenging.

Figure 10.3 shows the result of the reconstruction when perfect measures (with very accurate precision) are available. We use two different boundary potentials, $\psi = x_1$ and $\psi = x_2$. The initial guess is depicted on the left: it is equal to 1 inside the disk of radius 6 centered at the origin, and equal to the supposedly known conductivity $\gamma = 0.5$ near the boundary (outside the disk of radius 6). The two central pictures represent the collected data, $\mathcal{E}$ for $\psi = x_1$ on the left and $\mathcal{E}$ for $\psi = x_2$ on the right. Given the values of the contrast, we remark that although one can see the triangle and the L–shape inclusions on these plots, the circle is hardly noticeable. On the far right, the reconstructed conductivity is represented: it perfectly matches the target.

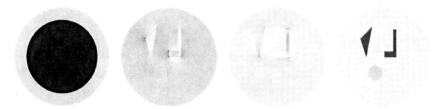

Fig. 10.3. Reconstruction test. From left to right, the initial guess, the collected data $\mathcal{E}$ (x_1 and x_2) and the reconstructed conductivity.

Bibliography and Discussion

The conductivity imaging technique called impediography, which is investigated in this chapter, was proposed in [5]. Motivated by the practical limitations of EIT, researches on impediography can be pursued in the following directions:

(i) Study the reconstruction capabilities of this method when only partial data, measured on a small portion of the boundary, is available.
(ii) Study the dependence of the algorithm on the global geometry of the body.
(iii) Study the sensitivity of the method to limitations on the intensities of the applied voltages, as electrical safety regulations limit the amount of the total current that patients can sustain.

Magnetic Resonance Elastography

Extensive work has been carried out in the past decade to image, by inducing motion, the elastic properties of human soft tissues. This wide application field, called elasticity imaging or elastography, is based on the initial idea that shear elasticity can be correlated with the pathological state of tissues.

Several techniques arose according to the type of mechanical excitation chosen (static compression, monochromatic, or transient vibration) and the way these excitations are generated (externally or internally). Different imaging modalities can be used to estimate the resulting tissue displacements.

Magnetic resonance elastography (MRE) is a new way of realizing the idea of elastography. It can directly visualize and quantitatively measure the displacement field in tissues subject to harmonic mechanical excitation at low-frequencies (10 to 1000 Hz). A phase-contrast MRI technique is used to spatially map and measure the complete three-dimensional displacement patterns. From this data, local quantitative values of shear modulus can be calculated and images that depict tissue elasticity or stiffness can be generated. The inverse problem for MRE is to determine the shape and the elastic parameters of an elastic anomaly from internal measurements of the displacement field. In most cases the most significant elastic parameter is the stiffness coefficient.

In this chapter, we combine the method of small volume expansions and a binary level set algorithm to solve the full three-dimensional inverse problem of the MRE.

11.1 Mathematical Model

Suppose that an elastic medium occupies a bounded domain Ω in $\mathbb{R}^3$, with a connected $\mathcal{C}^2$-boundary $\partial\Omega$. Let the constants (λ, μ) denote the Lamé coefficients of Ω, that are the elastic parameters in the absence of any anomalies and let the constant ρ denote the density of the background. Suppose that Ω contains an elastic anomaly D given by $D = \delta B + z$, where B is a bounded

$\mathcal{C}^2$-domain in $\mathbb{R}^3$. The domain B is considered to be a reference domain, the small number δ is the diameter of D, and z represents the location of D. Suppose that D has the pair of Lamé constants $(\tilde{\lambda}, \tilde{\mu})$ which is different from that of the background elastic body, (λ, μ), and let $\tilde{\rho}$ denote its density. It is always assumed that

$$\rho > 0, \ \mu > 0, \ 3\lambda + 2\mu > 0, \quad \tilde{\rho} > 0, \ \tilde{\mu} > 0 \text{ and } 3\tilde{\lambda} + 2\tilde{\mu} > 0 .$$

Consider the following transmission problem associated to the system of elastodynamics with the Dirichlet boundary condition:

$$\begin{cases} \displaystyle\sum_{j,k,l=1}^{3} \frac{\partial}{\partial x_j}\left(C_{ijkl} \frac{\partial u_k}{\partial x_l} \right) + \omega^2(\rho\chi(\Omega \setminus D) + \tilde{\rho}\chi(D))u_i = 0 \quad \text{in } \Omega, \\ \mathbf{u}\big|_{\partial\Omega} = \mathbf{g}, \end{cases} \tag{11.1}$$

for $i = 1, 2, 3$, where the elasticity tensor $C = (C_{ijkl})$ is given by

$$\begin{aligned} C_{ijkl} := &\left(\lambda\chi(\Omega \setminus D) + \tilde{\lambda}\chi(D) \right)\delta_{ij}\delta_{kl} \\ &+ \left(\mu\chi(\Omega \setminus D) + \tilde{\mu}\chi(D) \right)(\delta_{ik}\delta_{jl} + \delta_{il}\delta_{jk}) , \end{aligned} \tag{11.2}$$

$\omega > 0$ is the angular frequency of the mechanical oscillations, and u_i for $i = 1, 2, 3$, denote the components of the displacement field $\mathbf{u}$.

The Poisson ratios σ and $\tilde{\sigma}$ are given in terms of the Lamé parameters by

$$\sigma = \frac{\lambda/\mu}{1 + 2\lambda/\mu} \quad \text{and} \quad \tilde{\sigma} = \frac{\tilde{\lambda}/\tilde{\mu}}{1 + 2\tilde{\lambda}/\tilde{\mu}} . \tag{11.3}$$

It is known that in soft tissues, $\sigma, \tilde{\sigma} \approx 1/2$, or equivalently, $\lambda \gg \mu$ and $\tilde{\lambda} \gg \tilde{\mu}$. This makes it very difficult to estimate both parameters $\tilde{\mu}$ and $\tilde{\lambda}$ simultaneously.

From Sect. 7.6, the elasticity system (11.1) can be replaced with the modified Stokes system:

$$\begin{cases} (\mu\Delta + \omega^2\rho)\mathbf{u}_0 + \nabla p_0 = 0 \quad \text{in } \Omega \setminus \overline{D} , \\ (\tilde{\mu}\Delta + \omega^2\tilde{\rho})\mathbf{u}_0 + \nabla p_0 = 0 \quad \text{in } D , \\ \mathbf{u}_0\big|_- = \mathbf{u}_0\big|_+ \quad \text{on } \partial D , \\ (p_0|_+ - p_0|_-)\mathbf{N} + \mu\dfrac{\partial \mathbf{u}_0}{\partial \mathbf{N}}\bigg|_+ - \tilde{\mu}\dfrac{\partial \mathbf{u}_0}{\partial \mathbf{N}}\bigg|_- = 0 \quad \text{on } \partial D , \\ \nabla \cdot \mathbf{u}_0 = 0 \quad \text{in } \Omega , \\ \mathbf{u}_0 = \mathbf{g} \quad \text{on } \partial\Omega , \\ \displaystyle\int_\Omega p_0 = 0 . \end{cases} \tag{11.4}$$

Sect. 7.6.1 shows that the leading-order term in the displacement field perturbations that are due to the presence the elastic anomaly D is given by

$$\mathbf{u}_0(x) \approx \mathbf{U}_0(z) + \delta \hat{\mathbf{v}}_1(\frac{x-z}{\delta}) \quad \text{for } x \text{ near } z , \tag{11.5}$$

where $\mathbf{U}_0$ is the background field and $\hat{\mathbf{v}}_1$ is the unique solution to

$$
\begin{cases}
\mu \Delta \hat{\mathbf{v}}_1 + \nabla \hat{p}_0 = 0 & \text{in } \mathbb{R}^3 \setminus \overline{B} , \\
\tilde{\mu} \Delta \hat{\mathbf{v}}_1 + \nabla \hat{p}_0 = 0 & \text{in } B , \\
\hat{\mathbf{v}}_1|_- - \hat{\mathbf{v}}_1|_+ = 0 & \text{on } \partial B , \\
(\hat{p}_0 \mathbf{N} + \tilde{\mu} \frac{\partial \hat{\mathbf{v}}_1}{\partial \mathbf{N}})|_- - (\hat{p}_0 \mathbf{N} + \mu \frac{\partial \hat{\mathbf{v}}_1}{\partial \mathbf{N}})|_+ = 0 & \text{on } \partial B , \\
\nabla \cdot \hat{\mathbf{v}}_1 = 0 & \text{in } \mathbb{R}^3 , \\
\hat{\mathbf{v}}_1(\xi) - \nabla \mathbf{U}_0(z)\xi \to 0 & \text{as } |\xi| \to +\infty , \\
\hat{p}_0(\xi) \to 0 & \text{as } |\xi| \to +\infty .
\end{cases}
\tag{11.6}
$$

11.2 Binary Level Set Algorithm

Based on the inner asymptotic expansion (11.5) of $\delta \mathbf{u} := \mathbf{u}_0 - \mathbf{U}_0$, the perturbations in the displacement field that are due to the anomaly, we provide a reconstruction method of binary level set type.

The first step for the reconstruction procedure is to locate the anomaly. This can be done using the measurements $\delta \mathbf{u}$ of the perturbations in the displacement field far away from the anomaly. Suppose that z is reconstructed. Since the representation $D = z + \delta B$ is not unique, we can fix δ. We use a binary level set representation f of the scaled domain B:

$$f(x) = \begin{cases} 1, & x \in B , \\ -1, & x \in \mathbb{R}^3 \setminus \overline{B} . \end{cases}$$

Let

$$h(x) = \tilde{\mu}(f(\frac{x-z}{\delta}) + 1) - \mu(f(\frac{x-z}{\delta}) - 1) ,$$

and let β be a regularization parameter.

The second step is to fix a window W (for example a sphere containing z) and solve the following constrained minimization problem:

$$
\min_{\tilde{\mu}, f} L(f, \tilde{\mu}) = \frac{1}{2} \left\| \delta \mathbf{u}(x) - \delta \hat{\mathbf{v}}_1(\frac{x-z}{\delta}) + \nabla \mathbf{U}_0(z)(x-z) \right\|_{L^2(W)}^2 \\
+ \beta \int_W |\nabla h(x)| \, dx ,
\tag{11.7}
$$

subject to (11.6).

In the above, $\int_W |\nabla h| \, dx$ is the total variation of the shear modulus, and $|\nabla h|$ is understood as a measure:

$$\int_W |\nabla h| = \sup\left\{ \int_W h\nabla \cdot \mathbf{v} \, dx, \mathbf{v} \in \mathcal{C}_0^1(W) \text{ and } |\mathbf{v}| \leq 1 \text{ in } W \right\}.$$

This regularization indirectly controls both the length of the level set curves and the jumps in the coefficients.

The local character of the method is due to the decay of

$$\hat{\mathbf{v}}_1((\cdot - z)/\delta) - \nabla \mathbf{U}_0(z)(\cdot - z)/\delta$$

away from z. Replacing W by Ω in the above formulation does not lead to a better reconstruction of the shape and the shear modulus of the anomaly. This is one of the main features of the method.

The minimization problem (11.7) corresponds to a minimization with respect to $\tilde{\mu}$ followed by a step of minimization with respect to f. The minimization steps are over the set of $\tilde{\mu}$ and f and can be performed using a gradient based method with a line search. An augmented Lagrangian functional can be defined where the constraints given by (11.6) are incorporated. To find a discrete saddle point for this augmented Lagrangian functional, the Uzawa algorithm for variational binary level set methods can be used.

Of importance to us are the optimal bounds satisfied by the viscous moment tensor V. We should check for each step whether the bounds on V corresponding to (7.52) and (7.53) for $d = 3$ are satisfied. Set $\alpha = \mathrm{Tr}(V)$ and $\beta = \mathrm{Tr}(V^{-1})$ and suppose for simplicity that $\tilde{\mu} > \mu$. Then, these bounds can be rewritten (when $d = 3$) as follows:

$$\begin{cases} \alpha \leq 2(\tilde{\mu} - \mu)(3 + \dfrac{2\mu}{\tilde{\mu}})|D|, \\ \dfrac{2\mu(\tilde{\mu} - \mu)}{3\mu + 2\tilde{\mu}}|D| \leq \beta^{-1}. \end{cases}$$

In the case when they are not, we have to restate the value of $\tilde{\mu}$. Another way to deal with these bounds is to introduce them into the minimization problem (11.7) as a constraint.

Bibliography and Discussion

Several techniques for the estimation of soft tissue elasticity are currently being investigated. See for instance [107, 113, 105, 27, 28, 55].

MRE was first proposed in [101]. See also [95, 63, 116]. The results provided in this chapter are from [8]. In general, the viscoelastic parameters of biological tissues show anisotropic properties, i.e., the local value of elasticity is different in the different spatial directions [115]. It would be very interesting to extend the algorithm described in this chapter for detecting the shape and the anisotropic shear modulus of an anisotropic anomaly.

Recall that the main idea behind impediography (EIT by ultrasound focusing) is to create, by a non intrusive method, controlled perturbations inside the medium to be imaged, which in turn allow to reconstruct very accurately the unperturbed medium. Interestingly, it turns out that he same idea applies in elastic imaging. An ultrasound signal, focusing on a small spot localized at a position is applied to the medium to be imaged. The displacement field induced by the ultrasound wave is measured either inside the domain by an MRI system or on its surface. This new and promising imaging method is being developed at LOA. It offers a number of challenging mathematical problems to be solved.

References

1. R. Acharya, R. Wasserman, J. Stevens, and C. Hinojosa, Biomedical imaging modalities: a tutorial, Comput. Medical Imag. Graph., 19 (1995), 3–25.
2. R. Albanese and P.B. Monk, The inverse source problem for Maxwell's equations, Inverse Problems, 22 (2006), 1023–1035.
3. H. Ammari, An inverse initial boundary value problem for the wave equation in the presence of imperfections of small volume, SIAM J. Control Optim., 41 (2002), 1194–1211.
4. H. Ammari, G. Bao, and J. Flemming, An inverse source problem for Maxwell's equations in magnetoencephalography, SIAM J. Appl. Math., 62 (2002), 1369–1382.
5. H. Ammari, E. Bonnetier, Y. Capdeboscq, M. Tanter, and M. Fink, Electrical impedance tomography by elastic deformation, SIAM J. Appl. Math., to appear.
6. H. Ammari, P. Garapon, L. Guadarrama Bustos, and H. Kang, Transient anomaly imaging by the acoustic radiation force, preprint.
7. H. Ammari, R. Griesmaier, and M. Hanke, Identification of small inhomogeneities: asymptotic factorization, Math. of Comp., 76 (2007), 1425–1448.
8. H. Ammari, P. Garapon, H. Kang, and H. Lee, A method of biological tissues elasticity reconstruction using magnetic resonance elastography measurements, Quart. Appl. Math., 66 (2008), 139–175.
9. H. Ammari, E. Iakovleva, and D. Lesselier, Two numerical methods for recovering small electromagnetic inclusions from scattering amplitude at a fixed frequency, SIAM J. Sci. Comput., 27 (2005), 130–158.
10. H. Ammari, E. Iakovleva, and D. Lesselier, A MUSIC algorithm for locating small inclusions buried in a half-space from the scattering amplitude at a fixed frequency, Multiscale Model. Simul., 3 (2005), 597–628.
11. H. Ammari, E. Iakovleva, D. Lesselier, and G. Perrusson, A MUSIC-type electromagnetic imaging of a collection of small three-dimensional inclusions, SIAM J. Sci. Comput., 29 (2007), 674–709.
12. H. Ammari and H. Kang, High-order terms in the asymptotic expansions of the steady-state voltage potentials in the presence of conductivity inhomogeneities of small diameter, SIAM J. Math. Anal., 34 (2003), 1152–1166.
13. H. Ammari and H. Kang, *Reconstruction of Small Inhomogeneities from Boundary Measurements*, Lecture Notes in Mathematics, Vol. 1846, Springer-Verlag, Berlin, 2004.

14. H. Ammari and H. Kang, Boundary layer techniques for solving the Helmholtz equation in the presence of small inhomogeneities, J. Math. Anal. Appl., 296 (2004), 190–208.

15. H. Ammari and H. Kang, Reconstruction of elastic inclusions of small volume via dynamic measurements, Appl. Math. Opt., 54 (2006), 223–235.

16. H. Ammari and H. Kang, *Polarization and Moment Tensors: with Applications to Inverse Problems and Effective Medium Theory*, Applied Mathematical Sciences, Vol. 162, Springer-Verlag, New York, 2007.

17. H. Ammari, H. Kang, and H. Lee, A boundary integral method for computing elastic moment tensors for ellipses and ellipsoids, J. Comp. Math., 25 (2007), 2–12.

18. H. Ammari, H. Kang, G. Nakamura, and K. Tanuma, Complete asymptotic expansions of solutions of the system of elastostatics in the presence of an inclusion of small diameter and detection of an inclusion, J. Elasticity, 67 (2002), 97–129.

19. H. Ammari, O. Kwon, J.K. Seo, and E.J. Woo, Anomaly detection in T-scan trans-admittance imaging system, SIAM J. Appl. Math., 65 (2004), 252–266.

20. H. Ammari and J.K. Seo, An accurate formula for the reconstruction of conductivity inhomogeneities, Adv. Appl. Math., 30 (2003), 679–705.

21. S.R. Arridge, Optical tomography in medical imaging, Inverse Problems, 15 (1999), R41–R93.

22. M. Assenheimer, O. Laver-Moskovitz, D. Malonek, D. Manor, U. Nahliel, R. Nitzan, and A. Saad, The T-scan technology: Electrical impedance as a diagnostic tool for breast cancer detection, Physiol. Meas., 22 (2001), 1–8.

23. S. Baillet, J.C. Mosher, and R.M. Leahy, Electromagnetic brain mapping, IEEE Sign. Processing Magazine, Nov. 2001, 14–30.

24. G. Bal, Optical tomography for small volume absorbing inclusions, Inverse Problems, 19 (2003), 371–386.

25. D.C. Barber and B.H. Brown, Applied potential tomography, J. Phys. Sci. Instrum., 17 (1984), 723–733.

26. C. Bardos and M. Fink, Mathematical foundations of the time reversal mirror, Asymptot. Anal., 29 (2002), 157182.

27. J. Bercoff, M. Tanter, and M. Fink, Supersonic shear imaging: a new technique for soft tissue elasticity mapping, IEEE Trans. Ultrasonics, Ferro., Freq. Control, 51 (2004), 396–409.

28. J. Bercoff, M. Tanter, and M. Fink, The role of viscosity in the impulse diffraction field of elastic waves induced by the acoustic radiation force, IEEE Trans. Ultrasonics, Ferro., Freq. Control, 51 (2004), 1523–1536.

29. L. Borcea, G.C. Papanicolaou, C. Tsogka, and J.G. Berrymann, Imaging and time reversal in random media, Inverse Problems, 18 (2002), 1247–1279.

30. D. Brenner, J. Lipton, L. Kaufman, and S.J. Williamson, Somatically evoked magnetic fields of the human brain, Science, 199 (1978), 81–83.

31. W.L. Briggs and V.E. Henson, *The DFT: An Owner Manuel for the Discrete Fourier Transform*, SIAM, Philadelphia, 1995.

32. M. Brühl, M. Hanke, and M.S. Vogelius, A direct impedance tomography algorithm for locating small inhomogeneities, Numer. Math., 93 (2003), 635–654.

33. Y. Capdeboscq and H. Kang, Improved Hashin-Shtrikman bounds for elastic moment tensors and an application, preprint.

34. Y. Capdeboscq and M.S. Vogelius, A general representation formula for the boundary voltage perturbations caused by internal conductivity inhomogeneities of low volume fraction, Math. Modelling Num. Anal., 37 (2003), 159–173.

35. Y. Capdeboscq and M.S. Vogelius, Optimal asymptotic estimates for the volume of internal inhomogeneities in terms of multiple boundary measurements, Math. Modelling Num. Anal., 37 (2003), 227–240.

36. D.J. Cedio-Fengya, S. Moskow, and M.S. Vogelius, Identification of conductivity imperfections of small diameter by boundary measurements: Continuous dependence and computational reconstruction, Inverse Problems, 14 (1998), 553–595.

37. D.H. Chambers and J.G. Berryman, Analysis of the time-reversal operator for a small spherical scatterer in an electromagnetic field, IEEE Trans. Antennas and Propagation, 52 (2004), 1729–1738.

38. D.H. Chambers and J.G. Berryman, Time-reversal analysis for scatterer characterization, Phys. Rev. Lett., 92 (2004), 023902-1.

39. M. Cheney, The linear sampling method and the MUSIC algorithm, Inverse Problems, 17 (2001), 591–595.

40. M. Cheney and D. Isaacson, Distinguishability in impedance imaging, IEEE Trans. Biomed. Engr., 39 (1992), 852–860.

41. M. Cheney, D. Isaacson, and J.C. Newell, Electrical impedance tomography, SIAM Rev., 41 (1999), 85–101.

42. M. Cheney, D. Isaacson, J.C. Newell, S. Simske, and J. Goble, NOSER: an algorithm for solving the inverse conductivity problem, Int. J. Imag. Syst. Technol., 22 (1990), 66–75.

43. D. Colton and A. Kirsch, A simple method for solving inverse scattering problems in the resonance region, Inverse Problems, 12 (1996), 383–393.

44. D. Colton and R. Kress, *Inverse Acoustic and Electromagnetic Scattering Theory*, Applied Mathematical Sciences, Vol. 93, Springer-Verlag, New York, 1992.

45. G. Dassios, What is recoverable in the inverse magnetoencephalography problem?, Contemp. Math., 408 (2006), 181–200.

46. G. Dassios, A.S. Fokas, and F. Kariotou, On the non-uniqueness of the inverse MEG problem, Inverse Problems, 21 (2005), L1–L5.

47. G. Dassios and R.E. Kleinman, *Low Frequency Scattering*, Oxford Science Publications, The Clarendon Press, Oxford University Press, New York, 2000.

48. I. Daubechies, *Ten Lectures on Wavelets*, SIAM, Philadelphia, 1992.

49. A.J. Devaney, A filtered backpropagation algorithm for diffraction tomography, Ultrasonic Imaging, 4 (1982), 336–350.

50. A.J. Devaney, Time reversal imaging of obscured targets from multistatic data, IEEE Trans. Antennas Propagat., 523 (2005), 1600–1610.

51. A. El Badia and T. Ha-Duong, An inverse source problem in potential analysis, Inverse Problems, 16 (2000), 651–663.

52. H.W. Engl, M. Hanke, and A Neubauer, *Regularization of Inverse Problems*, Kluwer, Dordrecht, 1996.

53. L. Escauriaza and J.K. Seo, Regularity properties of solutions to transmission problems, Trans. Amer. Math. Soc., 338 (1) (1993), 405–430.

54. E. Fabes, C. Kenig, and G. Verchota, The Dirichlet problem for the Stokes system on Lipschitz domains, Duke Math. J., 57 (1988), 769–793.

55. J. Fehrenbach, M. Masmoudi, R. Souchon, and P. Trompette, Detection of small inclusions by elastography, Inverse Problems 22 (2006), 1055–1069.

56. M. Fink, Time-reversal acoustics in *Inverse Problems, Multi-Scale Analysis and Homogenization*, 151–179, edited by H. Ammari and H. Kang, Contemp. Math., Vol. 408, Rhode Island, Providence, 2006.

57. A.S. Fokas, I.M. Gel'fand, and Y. Kurylev, Inversion method for magnetoencephalography, Inverse Problems, 12 (1996), L9–L11.

58. A.S. Fokas, Y. Kurylev, and V. Marinakis, The unique determination of neural currents in the brain via magnetoencephalography, Inverse Problems, 20 (2004), 1067–1082.

59. G.B. Folland, *Introduction to Partial Differential Equations*, Princeton University Press, Princeton, NJ, 1976.

60. J.P. Fouque, J. Garnier, G. Papanicolaou, and K. Solna, *Wave Propagation and Time Reversal in Randomly Layered Media*, Springer-Verlag, New York, 2007.

61. A. Friedman and M.S. Vogelius, Identification of small inhomogeneities of extreme conductivity by boundary measurements: a theorem on continuous dependence, Arch. Rat. Mech. Anal., 105 (1989), 299–326.

62. D. Gisser, D. Isaacson, and J.C. Newell, Electric current tomography and eigenvalues, SIAM J. Appl. Math., 50 (1990), 1623–1634.

63. J.F. Greenleaf, M. Fatemi, and M. Insana, Selected methods for imaging elastic properties of biological tissues, Annu. Rev. Biomed. Eng., 5 (2003), 57–78.

64. C. Hazard and K. Ramdani, Selective acoustic focusing using time-harmonic reversal mirrors, SIAM J. Appl. Math., 64 (2004), 1057–1076.

65. S. Helgason, *The Radon Transform*, Progress in Mathematics, Vol. 5, Second Edition, Birkhäuser, 1999.

66. D. Holder, *Clinical and Physiological Applications of Electrical Impedance Tomography*, UCL Press, London, 1993.

67. Y. Huo, R. Bansal, and Q. Zhu, Modeling of noninvasive microwave characterization of breast tumors, IEEE Trans. Biomedical Eng., 51 (2004), 1089–1094.

68. M. Hämäläinen, R. Hari, R. Ilmoniemi, J. Knuutila, and O. Lounasmaa, Magnetoencephalography. Theory, instrumentation and application to noninvasive study of humain brain function, Rev. Mod. Phys., 65 (1993), 413–497.

69. D. Isaacson, Distinguishability of conductivities by electric current computed tomography, IEEE Trans. Medical Imag., 5 (1986), 91–95.

70. D. Isaacson and M. Cheney, Effects of measurements precision and finite numbers of electrodes on linear impedance imaging algorithms, SIAM J. Appl. Math., 51 (1991), 1705–1731.

71. D. Isaacson and E.L. Isaacson, Comments on Calderón's paper: "On an inverse boundary value problem", Math. Compt., 52 (1989), 553–559.

72. V. Isakov, *Inverse Source Problems*, AMS, Providence, RI, 1990.

73. V. Isakov, *Inverse Problems for Partial Differential Equations*, Applied Mathematical Sciences, Vol. 127, Springer-Verlag, New York, 1998.

74. J. Kaipio and E. Somersalo, *Statistical and Computational Inverse Problems*, Applied Mathematical Sciences, Vol. 160, Springer-Verlag, New York, 2005.

75. H. Kang and J.K. Seo, Layer potential technique for the inverse conductivity problem, Inverse Problems, 12 (1996), 267–278.

76. H. Kang and J.K. Seo, Identification of domains with near-extreme conductivity: Global stability and error estimates, Inverse Problems, 15 (1999), 851–867.

77. H. Kang and J.K. Seo, Inverse conductivity problem with one measurement: Uniqueness of balls in R^3, SIAM J. Appl. Math., 59 (1999), 1533–1539.

78. H. Kang and J.K. Seo, Recent progress in the inverse conductivity problem with single measurement, in *Inverse Problems and Related Fields*, CRC Press, Boca Raton, FL, 2000, 69–80.

79. O.D. Kellogg, *Foundations of Potential Theory*, Dover, New York, 1953.

80. Y.J. Kim, O. Kwon, J.K. Seo, and E.J. Woo, Uniqueness and convergence of conductivity image reconstruction in magnetic resonance electrical impedance tomography, Inverse Problems, 19 (2003), 1213–1225.

81. S. Kim, O. Kwon, J.K. Seo, and J.R. Yoon, On a nonlinear partial differential equation arising in magnetic resonance electrical impedance imaging, SIAM J. Math. Anal., 34 (2002), 511–526.

82. A. Kirsch, *An Introduction to the Mathematical Theory of Inverse Problems*, Applied Mathematical Sciences, Vol. 120, Springer-Verlag, New York, 1996.

83. A. Kirsch, The MUSIC algorithm and the factorisation method in inverse scattering theory for inhomogeneous media, Inverse Problems, 18 (2002), 1025–1040.

84. V. Kolehmainen, M. Lassas, and P. Ola, The inverse conductivity problem with an imperfectly known boundary, SIAM J. Appl. Math., 66 (2005), 365–383.

85. V.D. Kupradze, *Potential Methods in the Theory of Elasticity*, Daniel Davey & Co., New York, 1965.

86. O. Kwon and J.K. Seo, Total size estimation and identification of multiple anomalies in the inverse electrical impedance tomography, Inverse Problems, 17 (2001), 59–75.

87. O. Kwon, J.K. Seo, and J.R. Yoon, A real-time algorithm for the location search of discontinuous conductivities with one measurement, Comm. Pure Appl. Math., 55 (2002), 1–29.

88. O. Kwon, E.J. Woo, J.R. Yoon, and J.K. Seo, Magnetic resonance electrical impedance tomography (MREIT): simulation study of J -substitution algorithm IEEE Trans. Biomed. Eng., 49 (2002), 160–167.

89. O. Kwon, J.R. Yoon, J.K. Seo, E.J. Woo, and Y.G. Cho, Estimation of anomaly location and size using impedance tomography, IEEE Trans. Biomed. Engr., 50 (2003), 89–96.

90. O.A. Ladyzhenskaya, *The mathematical Theory of Viscous Incompressible Flow*, Second English Edition, Gordon and Breach, New York, 1969.

91. Z.P. Liang and P.C. Lauterbur, *Principle of Magnetic Resonance Principles*, IEEE Press Series in Biomedical Engineering, SPIE Press, New York, 2000.

92. R. Lipton, Inequalities for electric and elastic polarization tensors with applications to random composites. J. Mech. Phys. Solids, 41 (1993), 809–833.

93. J.J. Liu, H.C. Pyo, J.K. Seo, and E.J. Woo, Convergence properties and stability issues in MREIT algorithm, Contemp. Math., 408 (2006), 201–218.

94. S. Mallat, *A Wavelet Tour of Signal Processing*, Academic Press, San Diego, 1998.

95. A. Manduca, T.E. Oliphant, M.A. Dresner, J.L. Mahowald, S.A. Kruse, E. Amromin, J.P. Felmlee, J.F. Greenleaf, and R.L. Ehman, Magnetic resonance elastography: non-invasive mapping of tissue elasticity, Medical Image Analysis, 5 (2001), 237–254.

96. A. Markoe, *Analytic Tomography*, Encyclopedia of Mathematics and its Applications, Vol. 106, Cambridge University Press, Cambridge, 2006.

97. T.D. Mast, A. Nachman, and R.C. Waag, Focusing and imagining using eigenfunctions of the scattering operator, J. Acoust. Soc. Am., 102 (1997), 715–725.

98. W. McLean, *Strongly Elliptic Systems and Boundary Integral Equations*, Cambridge University Press, Cambridge, 2000.

99. C.M. Michel, M.M. Murray, G. Lantz, S. Gonzalez, L. Spinelli, and R. Grave de Peralta, EEG source imaging, Clinical Neurophys., 115 (2004), 2195–2222.

100. G.W. Milton, *The Theory of Composites*, Cambridge Monographs on Applied and Computational Mathematics, Cambridge University Press, 2001.
101. R. Muthupillai, D.J. Lomas, P.J. Rossman, J.F. Greenleaf, A. Manduca, and R.L. Ehman, Magnetic resonance elastography by direct visualization of propagating acoustic strain waves, Science, 269 (1995), 1854–1857.
102. F. Natterer, *The Mathematics of Computerized Tomography*, Classics in Applied Mathematics, SIAM, Philadelphia, 2001.
103. F. Natterer and F. Wübbeling, *Mathematical Methods in Image Reconstruction*, SIAM Monographs on Mathematical Modeling and Computation, SIAM, Philadelphia, 2001.
104. J.C. Nédélec, *Acoustic and Electromagnetic Equations. Integral Representations for Harmonic Problems*, Applied Mathematical Sciences, Vol. 144, Springer-Verlag, New-York, 2001.
105. K. Nightingale, M.S. Soo, R. Nightingale, and G. Trahey, Acoustic radiation force impulse imaging: In vivo demonstration of clinical feasibility, Ultrasound Med. Biol., 28 (2002), 227–235.
106. H.J. Nussbaumer, *Fast Fourier Transform and Convolution Algorithms*, Springer-Verlag, New York, 1982.
107. J. Ophir, I. Cespedes, H. Ponnekanti, Y. Yazdi, X. Li, Elastography: a quantitative method for imaging the elasticity of biological tissues, Ultrason. Imag., 13 (1991), 111–134.
108. I.G. Petrovsky, *Lectures on Partial Differential Equations*, Dover, New York, 1954.
109. C. Prada and M. Fink, Eigenmodes of the time-reversal operator: A solution to selective focusing in multiple-target media, Wave Motion, 20 (1994), 151163.
110. C. Prada, J.-L. Thomas, and M. Fink, The iterative time reversal process: Analysis of the convergence, J. Acoust. Soc. Amer., 97 (1995), 62–71.
111. F. Santosa and M.S. Vogelius, A backprojection algorithm for electrical impedance imaging, SIAM J. Appl. Math., 50 (1990), 216–243.
112. J. Sarvas, Basic mathematical and electromagnetic concepts of the biomagnetic inverse problem, Phys. Med. Biol., 32 (1987), 11–22.
113. A.P. Sarvazyan, O.V. Rudenko, S.D. Swanson, J.B. Fowlkes, and S.Y. Emelianov, Shear wave elasticity imagingA new ultrasonic technology of medical diagnostic, Ultrasound Med. Biol., 20 (1998), 1419–1436.
114. J.K. Seo, O. Kwon, H. Ammari, and E.J. Woo, Mathematical framework and anomaly estimation algorithm for breast cancer detection using TS2000 configuration, IEEE Trans. Biomedical Engineering, 51 (2004), 1898–1906.
115. R. Sinkus, M. Tanter, S. Catheline, J. Lorenzen, C. Kuhl, E. Sondermann, and M. Fink, Imaging anisotropic and viscous properties of breast tissue by magnetic resonance-elastography, Mag. Res. Med., 53 (2005), 372–387.
116. R. Sinkus, M. Tanter, T. Xydeas, S. Catheline, J. Bercoff, and M. Fink, Viscoelastic shear properties of in vivo breast lesions measured by MR elastography, Mag. Res. Imag., 23 (2005), 159–165.
117. E. Somersalo, M. Cheney, and D. Isaacson, Existence and uniqueness for electrode models for electric current computed tomography, SIAM J. Appl. Math., 52 (1992), 1023–1040.
118. M.E. Taylor, *Partial Differential Equations I. Basic Theory*, Applied Mathematical Sciences, Vol. 115, Springer-Verlag, New York, 1996.
119. C.W. Therrien, *Discrete Random Signals and Statistical Signal Processing*, Englewood Cliffs, NJ, Prentice-Hall, 1992.

120. M.S. Vogelius and D. Volkov, Asymptotic formulas for perturbations in the electromagnetic fields due to the presence of inhomogeneities, Math. Model. Numer. Anal., 34 (2000), 723–748.

121. A. Webb, *Introduction to Biomedical Imaging*, IEEE Press Series in Biomedical Engineering, Wiley-Interscience, New Jersey, 2003.

122. C.H. Wolters, L. Grasedyck, and W. Hackbusch, Efficient computation of lead field bases and influence matrix for the FEM- based EEG and MEG inverse problem, Inverse Problems, 20 (2004), 1099–1116.

123. C.H. Wolters, H. Koestler, C. Moeller, J. Härdtlein, L. Grasedyck, and W. Hackbusch, Numerical mathematics of the subtraction method for the modeling of a current dipole in EEG source reconstruction using finite element head models, preprint.

124. E.J. Woo, J.G. Webster, and W.J. Tompkins, A robust image reconstruction algorithm and its parallel implementation in electrical impedance tomography, IEEE Trans. Med. Imag., 12 (1993), 137–146.

125. C.C. Wood, Application of dipole localization methods to source identification of human evoked potentials, Ann. New York Acad. Sci., 388 (1982), 139–155.

126. T. Yorkey, J. Webster, and W. Tompkins, Comparing reconstruction algorithms for electrical impedance tomography, IEEE Trans. Biomed. Engr., 34 (1987), 843–852.

Index

Déjà parus dans la même collection

39. B. YCART : Modèles et algorithmes Markoviens. 2002

40. B. BONNARD, M. CHYBA : Singular Trajectories and their Role in Control Theory. 2003

41. A. TSYBAKOV : Introdution à l'estimation non-paramétrique. 2003

42. J. ABDELJAOUED, H. LOMBARDI : Méthodes matricielles – Introduction à la complexité algébrique. 2004

43. U. BOSCAIN, B. PICCOLI : Optimal Syntheses for Control Systems on 2-D Manifolds. 2004

44. L. YOUNES : Invariance, déformations et reconnaissance de formes. 2004

45. C. BERNARDI, Y. MADAY, F. RAPETTI : Discrétisations variationnelles de problèmes aux limites elliptiques. 2004

46. J.-P. FRANÇOISE : Oscillations en biologie : Analyse qualitative et modèles. 2005

47. C. LE BRIS : Systèmes multi-échelles : Modélisation et simulation. 2005

48. A. HENROT, M. PIERRE : Variation et optimisation de formes : Une analyse géometric. 2005

49. B. BIDÉGARAY-FESQUET : Hiérarchie de modèles en optique quantique : De Maxwell-Bloch à Schrödinger non-linéaire. 2005

50. R. DÁGER, E. ZUAZUA : Wave Propagation, Observation and Control in $1-d$ Flexible Multi-Structures. 2005

51. B. BONNARD, L. FAUBOURG, E. TRÉLAT : Mécanique céleste et contrôle des véhicules spatiaux. 2005

52. F. BOYER, P. FABRIE : Eléments d'analyse pour l'étude de quelques modèles d'écoulements de fluides visqueux incompressibles. 2005

53. E. CANCÈS, C. L. BRIS, Y. MADAY : Méthodes mathématiques en chimie quantique. Une introduction. 2006

54. J-P. DEDIEU : Points fixes, zeros et la methode de Newton. 2006

55. P. LOPEZ, A. S. NOURI : Théorie élémentaire et pratique de la commande par les régimes glissants. 2006

56. J. COUSTEIX, J. MAUSS : Analyse asympotitque et couche limite. 2006

57. J.-F. DELMAS, B. JOURDAIN : Modèles aléatoires. 2006

58. G. ALLAIRE : Conception optimale de structures. 2007

59. M. ELKADI, B. MOURRAIN : Introduction à la résolution des systèmes polynomiaux. 2007

60. N. CASPARD, B. LECLERC, B. MONJARDET : Ensembles ordonnés finis : concepts, résultats et usages. 2007

61. H. PHAM : Optimisation et contrôle stochastique appliqués à la finance. 2007

62. H. AMMARI : An Introduction to Mathematics of Emerging Biomedical Imaging. 2008

63. C. GAETAN, X. GUYON : Modélisation et statistique spatiales. 2008

Printed in the United Kingdom
by Lightning Source UK Ltd.
133323UK00001B/2/P